THE HOLISTIC GREEK DIET & WAY OF LIFE
A MODERNIZED LOOK AT THE ANCIENT MEDITERRANEAN DIET

YOTA KOUYAS GERRIOR R.H.N

The Holistic Greek Diet & Way of Life

A Modernized Look at the Ancient Mediterranean Diet

Yota Kouyas Gerrior R.H.N.

© **Copyright 2022 - All rights reserved.**

The content contained within this book may not be reproduced, duplicated or transmitted without direct written permission from the author or the publisher. Under no circumstances will any blame or legal responsibility be held against the publisher, or author, for any damages, reparation, or monetary loss due to the information contained within this book, either directly or indirectly. Legal Notice:

This book is copyright protected. It is only for personal use. You cannot amend, distribute, sell, use, quote or paraphrase any part, or the content within this book, without the consent of the author or publisher. Disclaimer Notice:

Please note the information contained within this document is for educational and entertainment purposes only. All effort has been executed to present accurate, up-to-date, reliable, complete information. However, no warranties of any kind are declared or implied. Readers acknowledge that the author is not engaged in rendering legal, financial, medical or professional advice. The content within this book has been derived from various sources. Please consult a licensed professional before attempting any techniques outlined in this book.By reading this document, the reader agrees that under no circumstances is the author responsible for any losses, direct or indirect, incurred due to the use of the information contained within this document, including, but not limited to, errors, omissions, or inaccuracies.

CONTENTS

Introduction	v
1. Holistic Nutrition—What It Means and Where It Began	1
2. Ancient Greek Diet vs Modern Greek Diet	14
3. How to Implement the Greek/Mediterranean Diet Today	30
4. Benefits of a Greek Holistic Diet/Mediterranean Plan	47
5. Greek Diet and Its Benefits to Various Body Systems	64
6. Olive Oil and Its Ancient Greek History	83
7. A Brief History of the Greeks and Their Love of Coffee	101
8. Greek Holistic Health With Herbs	118
Recipes	135
Afterword	141
About the Author	153
Also by Yota Kouyas Gerrior R.H.N	155

INTRODUCTION

In today's busy lifestyle and a demanding world, we all prefer convenience over anything, and that includes our eating habits. When we get hungry, we find it easier to order takeaway, open a can, or just go out and eat instead of having fresh foods. However, holistic nutritionists state that as much as convenience appears favourable and easy on the pocket, it is not the best for your health. With the global rise of obesity and diseases like diabetes, the connection between your health and what you eat has gradually gained widespread attention. As a result, people approach holistic nutrition to feed and help nourish their bodies.

The Greeks have a long history of influence over different parts of the world, including the United States. For instance, the Greek Revival architectural style gained popularity at the turn of the 19th

INTRODUCTION

century. It remains a timeless architectural style. Just as the Greek Revival architecture evoked political ideology, the Greek holistic nutrition strengthens healthier living style by reviving old culinary practices. These customs involve cooking and eating from Mother Nature's richness while appreciating what matters. The holistic nutrition theory holds that one's health is a complicated interplay between chemical and physical, emotional and mental, social and spiritual components of one's lifestyle and being. As a result, holistic nutritionists view health and wellness from the aspect of the whole person. Holistic nutrition stresses health maintenance by considering each person differently, using knowledge about essential nutrition as an effective tool. Holistic health fully requires involving the person in their health process and recognizing their inner wisdom by educating them and aiding them in creating a path to optimum health.

Food was very significant in the Greek line of thinking. John Wilkins, a classicist, points out that "in the Odyssey, for example, good men are distinguished from bad and Greeks from foreigners partly in terms of how and what they ate. Herodotus identified people partly in terms of food and eating." (Wikipedia Contributors, 2019). Frugality enforced by the nation's climatic and geographic characteristics was considered virtuous until the 3rd century BC. The Greeks were not opposed to eating indulgences, but they preferred simplicity. Hesiod described his "flesh of a heifer fed in the woods" as the ideal way to end a day (Wikipedia Contributors, 2019). Despite this, Chrysippus says that the best supper was one provided for free. Gastronomical and culinary Research was scorned as a sign of eastern fatalism: the Persian Empire's residents were regarded as decadent people due to their rich tastes represented in their cuisine. Even the Greek authors relished the opportunity to describe the Achaemenid Great King and his court's meal.

I have always been fascinated by health and nutrition and how food impacts the human body. So when I came across the concept of holistic health and wellness a few years ago, I was instantly captivated. I was so impressed by the idea that I began to make changes in my lifestyle right away. As a result of my curiosity, I became a registered holistic nutritionist, and here we are. The term 'holistic' refers to looking at something as a whole rather than just its pieces. This is what holistic nutrition accomplishes. It treats each person as an individual unit and nourishes them according to their lifestyle, fitness, and environment. Holistic nutritionists believe that you must feed your body, mind, and soul to obtain optimum health.

Embracing this way of eating, and doing so with your own specific needs in mind, will leave you feeling energized, rejuvenated, and strong. You'll be eating for comprehensive health and wellness, as well as for balance. You are one of a kind. As a result, what you eat should be as well. Yes, healthy is healthy, but everybody is unique and may require more or less specific nutrients to achieve their ideal level of health. Of course, eating healthy is the aim, but what is beneficial for one person may not benefit another. Particularly when health circumstances, lifestyle, and environment are taken into account. Food may be used as medication, as more and more people are discovering. In addition, people are starting to use food to aid their recovery. This has yielded excellent outcomes on numerous occasions.

I'm not suggesting medicine is terrible or that you should never use it. On the contrary, treatment is essential, beneficial, and unavoidable. I'm suggesting that we shouldn't take medicine for every minor condition. People underestimate the benefits and drawbacks of food on our bodies, souls, and minds. We now consider what we perceive as 'normal,' even though certain things are not. For example, PMS, gas, and inflammation are all considered 'normal.' But in a nutshell, they are not. You shouldn't feel bloated after eating, and you shouldn't have excruciating cramps during or before your period. This is your body's method of alerting you to the fact that something isn't quite right. As some health concerns, such as obesity, heart problems, and anxiety, grow more common in our society, more individuals change to a holistic approach to recover their health.

Working as a researcher for holistic health and studying its nutritional aspects for more than ten years, I have learned a lot about how the Greek diet worked in ancient times. After I received my Diploma in Natural Health and Nutrition from The Canadian School of Natural Nutrition, I used the healthcare practices to help many individuals with chronic stressors through nutritional coaching. In all these years of nutritional coaching, I have realized how some simple holistic nutrition techniques can help energize your mind, body, and spirit and reduce fatigue. I have learned to reverse the negative aspects of stress and move towards a more positive outlook. Through this book, I want to share these techniques with you. This book will help you overcome your daily stressors by following a holistic approach to life. I believe in looking at the positive points in everything I do, and that has helped me turn my view of life into the most enjoyable version it can be. This book is the essence of what I have learned and practiced so far in my life.

In this book, together, we take a look back at and celebrate ancient Greek nutrition, which was abundant—full of colourful, fresh fruits and vegetables, fish, whole foods, nuts, and seeds baked into rich bread, and legumes for protein for the rest of the year. Today, we can gain the benefits of a half-

INTRODUCTION

century of study into Greek food and way of life. Several health benefits have been revealed due to this way of life. Ancient Greek food and lifestyle have been linked to increased vitality and a lower risk of stroke, cancer, heart disease, diabetes, Alzheimer's disease, arthritis, congenital disabilities, age-related blindness, asthma, and allergies. Ancel Keys, an American biologist, recognized that the men of Crete lived long, healthy, active lives in 1958 (Moore-Pastides, 2010). Keys was the first to chronicle the Mediterranean lifestyle and diet, coining the phrase "Mediterranean diet" in the process.

His main results were that the people of Crete lived longer due to their essential diet of olive oil, cereals (primarily bread), beans, fruits, and vegetables with smaller amounts of animal protein. Positive health necessitates understanding man's primary constitution and the effects of diverse diets. However, eating alone is not enough for good health (Moore-Pastides, 2010). There should also be exercise, the results of which must be recorded. The body will become ill if there is a lack of nourishment or activity. Holistic health focuses on the whole bodily system rather than a particular practice or therapy. Eating with purpose, also called intuitive eating or holistic eating, is essential for living a better, more aware life. Understanding the food sources, you're consuming and how they can affect your immunity, health, and other issues is an essential aspect of the holistic eating philosophy, emphasizing long-term sustenance. Both homeopaths and naturopaths believe that when our bodily systems are given the proper attention and care, they can help themselves by locating and resolving the fundamental cause of illness.

Practitioners of holistic medicine may aid with various medical ailments, such as improving cancer care with specific nutritional programs as part of mind-body medicine. Unprocessed, unulterated foods full of nutrients are the basic concepts of holistic nutrition, which is all about consuming healthy food as close to its original state as possible. According to holistic experts, food provides more than just sustenance for the body; it can act as medicine. Learning about your body and what it requires is crucial to following holistic nutrition concepts. Different people need various things. It depends on your biochemical composition and biological factors (Moore-Pastides, 2010).

We prefer to receive as much of our nutrients from food as possible; however, soil depletion affects the nutritional quality. There is no such thing as a "universal food supplement." The most successful technique is to use a customized diet program tailored to your specific biochemistry. Holistic nutrition is customized, personalized, and tailored to your requirements. It considers a person's entire physical and physiological well-being and the problems they attempt to resolve. It also examines the fundamental issues affecting your health and any disease or sickness you want to help to achieve the desired results. Varied ailments, disorders, and conditions have various nutritional needs, and each reacts differently to food and nutrition.

If you are new to holistic nutrition, it's usually better to start small and slowly make changes so that they don't appear so drastic and challenging to maintain. Be gentle and nice to yourself while simultaneously exercising self-control. It takes time and effort to change. You will also want to keep track of how you feel and adapt to changes, so if you implement too many changes at once, you won't be able to tell which actions have given you the most benefits. Your demands may vary over time due to current health practices or failures, and you may need to modify your diet accordingly. You can never be wrong with holistic nutrition, no matter your position or condition. It enhances the level of efficiency and a better standard of living. Your mental, bodily, and spiritual well-being will be more balanced and harmonious.

1
HOLISTIC NUTRITION—WHAT IT MEANS AND WHERE IT BEGAN

Traditional cuisine is such an essential element of learning about a country. If you have visited Greece, you undoubtedly still remember the unusual tastes and flavours you experienced. If you haven't already, it's most likely one of several reasons you want to go. Hippocrates said, "Let food be thy medicine, and let medicine be thy food," and he was not wrong (Welch, 2021). The Greek diet is considered one of the greatest diets of all because it precisely showcases the concept of "you are what you eat." Apart from a few distinctions, this diet is similar in several countries across the Mediterranean. Therefore, the "Greek diet" is generally categorized under a broad range of the "Mediterranean diet." In this chapter, you will learn what made the Greek diet a source of holistic nutrition and how it became one of the ideal eating methods for people.

All About Holistic **Nutrition**

The term "holistic health" has a range of meanings in literature: A meaningful spiritual practice, a happy career, regular physical activity, and strong interpersonal connections, to name a few. Holism comes from the Greek term holos, which means 'whole.' Holism is not a religion or cult; instead, it is a way of thinking that considers everything in its entirety. Jan Smuts initially used it in his book *Holism and Evolution* in 1926. Holistic health usually comprises the whole person's body, mind, and spirit. A holistic approach to treatment entails more than simply eliminating symptoms. The ancient Greeks recognized the importance of physical and social circumstances and individual conduct in maintaining good health. They described health as a condition of external and internal dynamic equilibrium. They also considered the social and physical aspects of health, the empowerment of communities and individuals through modern democratic and collaborative institutions, and a focus on wellness training and skill development. They also understood the value of supporting conditions and effective public policies and reshaped medicine to be more natural and humane. A clean diet centred on nutritious, seasonal, and fresh foods free of chemicals, such as a spectrum of fruits and vegetables, healthy fats, and much more plant-based proteins, including those found in cereals, grains, and seeds, is recommended by holistic nutrition. Eggs, fish, meats, and dairy products are also included in some diets.

IN HOLISTIC HEALTH, there are three significant medical customs. They are as follows:

- Ayurveda: Ayurveda is an ancient Indian medical tradition. Ayurveda can be traced back to a text authored in the 6th century BC by Sushruta, the "Father of Surgery." The therapeutic method is based on beliefs in the universe's five major elements, the body's seven primary components, and the three' doshas,' or biological forces, that each represents. Ayurvedic holistic practitioners educate their patients to find balance and moderation using an eight-part treatment system.
- Herbal medicine: Herbal medicine is the most ancient kind of health care accessible to humankind, and it promotes overall balance. Indigenous peoples have used plant medicinal properties worldwide and

throughout history. TCM and Ayurveda both rely heavily on herbal medicine.
- Western herbalism: It focuses on the medical properties of plants and herbs. It originated in ancient Greece before spreading throughout Europe and North and South America.

Holistic health practitioners use a variety of approaches to helping the body, but they all follow the same core principles. They follow the traditional belief that one's health is most beneficial when the whole person is considered instead of specific symptoms, body parts, or ailments. As Socrates stated in the 4th century BC, "the part can never be well unless the whole is well" (NutritionBreathroughs.com, 2016). Holistic health is a condition of equilibrium, not just the absence of illness. Holistic health training teaches the interdependence of mind, body, soul, and the surroundings, just like it has for the past several thousand years.

What Hippocrates Taught Us

Asclepius and Hippocrates, as represented in the Hippocratic Oath, centred medical practice on the holistic approach and treatment of illnesses, emphasizing the importance of correctly understanding the patient's medical condition, independence, and the need for balance between the personal, social, and natural surroundings. Hippocrates (ca. 460–370 BC), an ancient physician, developed health principles more profoundly. Hippocrates' corpus, which consists of about 60 works, was most likely produced by several authors, including Hippocrates himself and his followers, who built the foundations of medical science (Kleisiaris et al., 2014). As per the pioneering text "On Airs, Waters, and Places," the Hippocratic school's most significant contribution to medical science, the definition of health is based on an equilibrium attained between environmental factors on the one side (temperature, wind, water, food, and ground) and personal habits on the other side (alcohol, diet, sexual behaviour, leisure, and work) (Tountas, 2017). The' internal' equilibrium of the four physiological fluids is determined by an individual's external' equilibrium with their surroundings. As per the literature, the essential concept of the Hippocratic philosophy was "a healthy mind in a healthy body." The Hippocratic delivery of care was divided into three categories: promoting health, intervening trauma care, and mental health and art therapy interventions (Kleisiaris et al., 2014).

Physical activity was promoted as an essential aspect of overall health, and the relevance of nutrition was emphasized in improving performance during the Olympic Games. Hippocrates pioneered surgical procedures used in trauma care, owing to the numerous wars in ancient Greece (Kleisiaris et al., 2014). The earliest categorization of mental diseases, proposed by Hippocrates, was followed by cognitive treatment and art therapy interventions. Music and drama were implemented as management techniques in treating the illness and improving human behaviour in this category. The Hippocratic concept of health care provision was based on a comprehensive approach to health care, with standards and ethical guidelines still in effect today. The Hippocratic tradition focused on environmental factors and helping with diseases. They emphasized the importance of psychological factors, lifestyle and nutrition, independence of spirit, mind, body, and balance between a person and the surroundings. The Hippocratic physicians ensured the patient was healthy.

The Pathogenic Process

According to Hippocrates, the pathogenic process is caused by overturning equilibrium and dominating any of the four fluids, resulting in sickness (Tountas, 2017). The Hippocratic practitioner who came to treat the residents of a town had to examine not only the seasons, the temperatures, the water people used, and the geography of the area, but also the lifestyle they lived: If they drank a lot of wine, ate well, exercised regularly, got enough rest, and worked hard. The ancients emphasized the importance of a healthy diet. The Greek word diaita, on the other hand, referred to more than just food and drink; dietetica (dietetics), the foundation of health and wellness, comprised a complete lifestyle. The Hippocratic process proposed a natural explanation for sickness. Hippocrates, for example, made some statements about male impotence among the Scythians linked to factors like rheumatism, horse riding, sheer fatigue, weather and ground conditions, and dietary patterns (Tountas, 2017).

How the Environment **Affects Us**

Since ancient times, humans have learned to adapt to the surroundings in which they live to survive, which implies that we look out for factors in the environment that are in our favour. For example, we look for safety and security wherever we live and find physical and psychological comfort. The retailers and other industries understand what we want and create a favourable atmosphere with safety, entertainment, and healthcare amenities.

BELOW ARE a few examples of what effect the environment has on an individual:

- The environment can encourage or discourage social interaction, thereby impacting social support.
- The environment can influence a person's behaviour and actions.
- It can influence a person's mood. For instance, bright lights can energize a person, while dim lights can do the opposite.

As per Hippocraties, winds significantly influence the health of an individual. He stated, "Cities faced towards the sunrise are healthier than those which are faced towards the North and … warm winds" (Tountas, 2017). He further mentioned the significance of the political and social environment in his writings. The advent of democracy in ancient Greece led to the departure of the heteronomous status quo and started a new movement towards autonomy (Tountas, 2017). However, even before Greek democracy flourished, social conditions already affected health. The medical theorist and philosopher Alcmaeon emphasizes health as isonomy, the equality of rights, and the balance of forces in the human body, including fluids, bitter, dry, and sweet. Isonomy affects not only the health of the citizens but also democracy. On the other hand, monarchy leads to disease. It destroys a city and isonomy by forcing a single rule on everyone.

How Education and Empowerment Affect Your Health

According to today's Ottawa Charter, the central aspect for achieving social development skills is empowering people, both as a community and as individuals, which is accomplished mainly through supportive environments and health education (Tountas, 2017). Even though ancient Greek philosophy doesn't mention the term' empowerment,' the Greek intellect was focused around the liberty of individuals from the grips of superstition and ignorance, directing people towards self-sufficiency—this concept, closely connected to the current ideas of empowerment.

Self-sufficiency is defined by philosopher Pythagoras as a state where a person is not dependent on others. Similarly, the followers of Pythagoras also emphasized self-maintained hygiene, also called the "Pythagorean way of life" (Tountas, 2017). Moderation, keeping oneself calm, and practicing self-control were keys to reaching a state of perfect health equilibrium. Diet, music, and gymnastics were used to restore health when it lost its equilibrium. Therefore, for a person to live as he should, there was a need for systematic preparatory education. Aristippus, a student of Socrates, promoted a theory based on the principle of self-sufficiency and encouraged the practice of life, which aimed to enjoy life as much as we can, given we are in control of our circumstances and our behaviours all the time. It was the time in the philosophical context that led to the emergence of health education (Tountas, 2017).

Ancient Ways Are Still Effective

Even though the scientific explanation for the importance of physical activity and diet for health and well-being is a modern phenomenon, the ancient Greeks were aware of this essential link. According to current research, regular exercise and a wholesome diet are unquestionably necessary for one's long-term well-being. But on the other hand, inadequate exercise is not only harmful to the body's overall processes, but it also leads to a number of chronic health problems, including colon cancer, Type 2 diabetes, coronary heart disease, and ischemic stroke, etc.

For their Empires, the Greeks needed to be in excellent form. Fitness was a cornerstone of military prowess. In Ancient Greek regions, children were encouraged and obliged to be active. Physical training was utilized to instill discipline, mental tenacity, and the value of good health among young Spartans. Men joined the Spartan army just at 13 and stayed until they were 60. In war, being unfit meant injury or worse. The outcomes were self-evident.

Hippocrates was the first to propose the innovative idea that diseases are caused by either consuming too much food or doing too much physical activity—when the two are balanced, they produce excellent health results. In his first book, *On Dietetics*, he writes that healthy eating alone will not keep an individual healthy; he must also engage in physical activity. While nutrition and exercise have diametrically opposed qualities, they contribute to good health. Exercise can deplete the body's components, while food and drink can replenish them. It appears that determining the specific capabilities of various activities, both natural and artificial, and which one of them helps in muscle development is essential.

Furthermore, exercise must be regulated to the amount of food consumed, the individual's propensity, age, the period of the year, the changing winds, the geographical location in which the individual lives, and the weather conditions of the particular year. People ate fresh cheese, veggies, and meat in prehistoric days. Their diet was high in protein, whole grains, and healthy fats. They lacked refrigerators and freezers. They ate just fresh food or nothing at all. They ate rich foods grown on the ground and animals bred on the plains.

Our bodies are built to move, and despite overwhelming evidence of the benefits of regular physical activity, most people spend very little time moving at work, at home, or during transportation and leisure activities. Regular calorie burn for urban people is projected to have fallen by roughly 800 kcal during the final half of the twentieth century, similar to daily walking of around 15 km. Sedentary behaviour is so pervasive in modern culture that it has achieved epidemic levels, posing a threat to health and well-being.

No matter how great or life-changing a specific diet may be, adopting a new eating pattern is always challenging. Everybody has particular eating habits and patterns, favouring foods that may or may not taste good or make people feel better simply because we've taken a liking to it and the customs surrounding it. Most people who try to implement a whole new eating style and intend to stick with it ultimately fail after only a few days. If you already eat mainly packaged, processed, and quick meals, or if you only eat a few Pillar Foods, you should begin the Greek diet with baby steps, modifying one or two items as to what you eat or drink for at least a week. For example, for starters, quit drinking soda and replace it with a cup of coffee as your daily energy drink. You'll be ready to adopt the diet as a whole once you've removed most of the packaged foods from your daily consumption and attempt to incorporate more of the Pillar Foods. Pick a day to start the diet, preferably one that you don't work if you're employed: It may be simpler to stick to a new habit if you combine a new food plan with a work schedule.

2
ANCIENT GREEK DIET VS MODERN GREEK DIET

The Greeks like eating, and their passion for food is well-known worldwide. Their food is characterized by a wide range of flavours, aromas, smells, colours, and textures. Their cuisine is nutritious, tasty, and enjoyable to make. They're so enthusiastic about their cuisine that Archestratus, a Greek poet and food enthusiast, is also said to have created the first recipe book in 350 BC. We know that the ancient Greeks strove to build a civilized lifestyle that distinguished them from the barbarians and that food played an essential role in this process. Of course, animals and so-called barbarians ate together, but what made a meal' civilized' were explicit norms (for example, how to pour wine properly).

. . .

Breakfast

Breakfast for most ancient Greeks consisted of bread dipped in wine. It was known as akratisma in ancient Greece. The classic Greek breakfast consists of bread, cheese, and fresh fruits, with adults finishing with a cup of coffee. Bread soaked in wine was all the ancient Greeks ate. The bread was prepared from barley, the primary source of all bread. It was most likely hard to swallow. The Greeks would dip it in wine to soften it and make it easier to consume. The bread had a vital role in the Ancient Greek diet. Although it was frequently prepared at home, the Ancient Greeks were not afraid to be creative with their concoctions. According to one source from the Ancient Greek academic Athenaeus, there were 72 different varieties of bread, which is more than enough to equal the variety available today. Wheat-based bread was consumed by the wealthy Ancient Greeks, whereas barley-based bread was consumed by the poor. Pasteli is one of those dishes that has undoubtedly been there for a long time. In terms of eating habits, the ancient Greeks ate three times a day, much as we do now. They got up and ate breakfast, took a lunch break in the middle of the day, and finished the day with dinner and probably a little dessert as Greeks identified the downside of sugar.

Greeks also ate a pancake-like dish known as teganites. Teganites were supposedly a favourite breakfast food of the Ancient Greeks. Wheat flour, olive oil, honey, and curdled milk were used to make these pancake-like products. Even though they are no longer regarded as a morning staple, they are nevertheless a popular Greek meal. They are generally topped with honey or cheese and prepared with wheat flour, olive oil, honey, and curdled milk. While milk was occasionally given as medication, it was never drunk daily. Ancient Greeks did not use butter and cheese because of the negative impacts on the body. However, they mainly consumed goat's milk in these circumstances. If you want to eat like an Ancient Greek today, eliminate cow milk and heavy dairy products from your diet!

Lunch

Lunch was traditionally the primary meal of the day, especially in rural regions, and was eaten early in the afternoon. It followed a few hours of repose, during which people remained at home, and schools and businesses were closed. On the other hand, people nowadays have a light lunch with no specific midday breaks. They may have a large meal or wait till later to eat bread. Bread and wine were also served at this noon meal, but the Greeks drank the wine rather than just soaking their bread in it. Lunch was seen as a noon snack in Greece; therefore, figs, salted fish, cheeses, olives, and other bread were typical. Figs were an essential element of the daily diet in Ancient Greece, especially for the working class. They were eaten with other fruits, such as apples, and were reputedly used as a bread replacement. Greek islanders pressed the figs to modify the texture and make them stodgier. In the meanwhile, fig leaves were employed to wrap fish.

Dinner

In Greece, dinner was and continues to be the most substantial meal of the day. It was a time when everyone would get together with their friends—not family—to discuss philosophy or current affairs. Traditionally, men and women ate their meals apart. Enslaved persons in certain houses would serve the males first, then the women, and lastly themselves. If the household did not have enslaved labourers, the ladies of the home would serve the men first and then eat when the men were finished. The majority of the food eaten was during lunchtime. Eggs from quail and chickens, fish, legumes, olives, cheeses, bread, figs, and any vegetables they could cultivate, such as arugula, asparagus, cabbage, carrots, and cucumbers, were all eaten by the ancient Greeks.

The Three Pillars of Food

Bread, wine, and olive oil were the three most vital components for the Ancient Greeks. This was part of the dietary model, or food ideology, as it was called. Along with honey and figs, these delicacies signified frugality and the simple life for the Greeks. This represented patriotism because these basic meals were produced in Greece; therefore, they didn't need to import rare luxury delicacies because they were content with what they had. It was also supposed to have something to do with conquering territories where olives and vines flourished; they should be captured and become Greek wherever they grew.

Bread ('Deipnosophistae')

The *Deipnosophistae* (dinner table philosophers), often known as the earliest cookbook, emphasizes the significance of bread in ancient Greek culture. Bread served as an essential source of nutrition and health at the table (there were three daily meals). There were unique bread and pastries for all events, such as festivities, entertainment, and religious festivals. Coarse brown raised bread, produced from emmer wheat and barley, white bread made from refined flour, oven bread, bread cooked in ashes, and wafer bread, as well as soft pastries like barley cakes and sesame cake, were among the delicacies available. The bread was the table's centrepiece, accompanied by meat, fish, vegetables, and fruits.

The bread was called after ingredients, shape, baking methods, and provenance and rated on quality; the colour mattered, and white was favoured. By far, Athens was the most important city in Greece. The famed Athenian baker, Therion, was widely referenced in ancient literature and characterized as one of the body's marvellous caregivers. By far the most prosperous city was Athens. Baking bread was a typical family activity that required the participation of the women of the home and may take up to five hours each day.

On the other hand, commercial bakeries were prominent in the 5th century BC, and fresh bread could be purchased at the market. The ordinary Athenian consumed roughly 600 to 800 grams of bread per day, but bread also featured prominently in the diets of the rich. The Athenian high classes ate white bread, which was costly since wheat was imported, primarily from Egypt, because wheat growth in Mediterranean climes was difficult. The ancient Greeks worshipped Demeter, the Olympian goddess of agriculture, grain, and life-giving bread. The Greek practice of baking a tasty variety of freshly made bread dates back generations. The Greek Breakfast table includes village-style, white, and whole wheat bread, all freshly made.

The bread was and continues to be one of the

primary components of existence for the Greeks. That's why they offer alternate forms when they don't' knead' it. The most well-known is a pie made with flour and water to make pastry puffs out of whatever is available in the kitchen (depending on the season). Rusks were also an emergency option, as they could be stored for months and met the demands of mariners and artisans.

Wine

The wine was the ancient Greeks' primary beverage, aside from water. (The women of the home had to fetch water regularly.) The Greeks consumed the wine at all meals and throughout the day. They produced red, white, rose, and port wines, with Thassos, Lesbos, and Chios being the primary production locations. On the other hand, the ancient Greeks did not drink their wine directly since it was deemed savage. Instead, water was used to dilute the wine. The Greeks drank for the enjoyment of the drink, not to become inebriated. They also drank kykeon, a drink made from barley gruel, water (or wine), herbs, and goat cheese that had a shake consistency. Although the Romans had a reputation for being indulgent wine drinkers and grape eaters, the Ancient Greeks enjoyed wine just as much. It was a drink served with every meal, along with water.

The Ancient Greeks also traded it with their neighbours, where wine from the islands of Crete, Rhodes, and Levos was a prominent export. Great wineries that export globally may still be found in Greece. Wine is an integral part of every Grecian meal and has strong origins in Greek culinary history. The wine was first brought to Greece about 4000 BC, according to ancient texts, and has since become an essential component of Greek cuisine. The wine was viewed as a gift from the Gods, according to the texts, and considered a component of Greek agriculture. It was then drunk after being diluted with water. Dionysus, a legendary figure with the mind of a man and the nature of a beast, was honoured with wine-drinking celebrations.

Olive Oil

Olive oil is always present at the Greek table; this highly regarded oil is used in nearly every meal prepared by Greek chefs. A bottle is always on the table, as guests are encouraged to use it as a garnish on their dish right before eating. It's also worth noting that olive oil isn't just vital in Greece now; it also played a significant role in Ancient Greece. Olive oil was used on salads in Greece, although generally used in cooking. While other cultures used olive oil uncooked, primarily for sprinkling on salads or toast, Greeks consumed it in their cooking, sautéing, roasting, and frying. There was also a food category called lathera, which originates from the Greek word lathi, which means oil. The word directly translates to "oily" and refers to veggies that have been cooked in olive oil. It was commonly stated that one should not cook using olive oil for various reasons, including smoke point, the olive oil becoming cancerogenic, and a variety of other assertions.

According to tradition, Athena, the Goddess of Wisdom, bestowed the olive tree onto Athens as a gift. In certain versions of the myth, it's unclear if the olive tree was already present in other regions of Ancient Greece. However, the anecdote demonstrates that the olive tree was highly significant to Ancient Greeks. The Ancient Greeks recognized the nutritional value of olive oil. As a result, in the 7th century BC, leading philosophers and physicians in Ancient Greece investigated the use of olive oil as a medicine. When Hippocrates was treating his patients, he employed it for various purposes. Olive oil is now commonly used to help stomach issues, skin diseases, coughs, sore throats, congestion, and other respiratory problems.

It's also regarded as a vital aesthetic aid and used in helping overall health. The oil is used to help soothe irritated skin, tame frizzy hair, and battle dry skin. Olive oil is still widely used in Greece to help with wounds, sunburns, and other skin conditions.

It is also reported to be highly nutritious and beneficial to one's health.

The Ancient Greek Way of Eating

Ancient Greek diet was similar to what we eat now, but it lacked several ingredients that have become staples of modern Greek cuisine. Tomatoes, potatoes, peppers, and bananas did not appear in Greece until after the 15th-century arrival of the Americas because those products originated there. Oranges, lemons, eggplant, and rice were also delivered later. The foundation of the ancient Greek diet is legumes, vegetables, and fruit. However, as a coastal nation with several islands, seafood was a diet staple, while livestock farming and hunting provided meat and sport. Meat and seafood consumption varied according to the household's affluence and geography. Traditional ancient Greek meals included these components in different degrees and were prepared using various cooking methods to modify the look and taste. The frugality of ancient Greek cuisine reflected the hardships of agriculture. The old Greek diet was based on the Mediterranean trinity of olive oil, wheat, wine, and other foods available to the Greeks. Many ancient Greek recipes have survived to this day. Below is a breakdown of the types of foods the ancient Greeks had:

Pure Vegetarianism

Relying only on vegetarianism, on the other hand, was a well-known practice, with lentil soup or a gruel of barley boiled with cabbage leaves and turnips mentioned in the *Odyssey* and *Herodotus' Histories*. Another popular grain-based food recorded in Homer was kykeon, which consisted of barley cooked over an open fire with wine and goat's cheese. Humble rural and city dwellers would have supplemented their daily meals with vegetables, fruit, dry nuts, and maybe a goat or sheep milk, cheese, or oxygala, a type of yogurt. Warriors, according to Aristophanes, ate modest meals, often consisting simply of cheese and onions. Spartans, known for their austerity, made a black soup of blood and boiled pig's leg seasoned with vinegar, which they served with barley, wine, fruit, and raw vegetables.

Non-Vegeterian

The ancient Greeks recognized the health benefits of meat. They ate many roasted meats, mainly lamb, goat, or pig. However, meat intake was not as frequent in antiquity as today, with special feasts or occasional appearances in one's weekly or monthly schedule being the norm. Cows, birds (thrushes, doves, quails, blackbirds, geese), wild hair, and deer, among other animals, were presumably more common in the countryside than it was in the city. Eels, river/lake fish, and different other types of seafood (particularly fresh or dried/salted fish) were also everyday menu items. Less advantaged members of society and the priests had access to meat through religious offerings, which served as a crucial social redistribution mechanism.

Wine Discipline

The wine was never drunk 'straight,' but instead blended in big or small pots and poured from a pitcher into the guest's drinking cup. The host was in charge of allocating the wine and preventing over-intoxication, which helped avoid excessive drunkenness, which was extensively mocked in Greek comic plays and was considered a hallmark of 'barbarian' foreign civilizations (at least by the elite).

SELECTION OF FOOD

Meats, vegetables, and fruit were delicately picked, cooked, and frequently served in two courses. While a simple supper would finish with cooked chickpeas, fresh or dried beans, apples, or figs. Archestratus recommends avoiding these at an expensive symposium instead of serving a delightful

Athenian cheesecake or at the very least one covered with Attica's excellent honey.

EXTENDING **Hospitality**

The ancient Greeks aspired to build a civilized lifestyle that distinguished them from the barbarians, and food played a vital role in this process. Animals and so-called barbarians also ate together, but what defined a meal as' civilized' were explicit norms (for example, the appropriate manner to pour wine) and sociability (eating and drinking with good company). Food and eating were not only required to meet bodily necessities but also a social occasion for Greeks.

Modern Greek Diet

Since ancient times, Greek food has been regarded as one of the most significant in the world. In truth, fashionable notions such as farm-to-table have long been a part of their society, while not exactly a Greek innovation. The Greek diet is a Mediterranean-style diet that emphasizes fresh fruits and vegetables, cheese, eggs, seafood, and meat. Greeks use plenty of olive oil since it is a healthier alternative to other oils. The well-known Greek salad has a lot of olive oil, onions, Greek tomatoes, and feta cheese. Tzatziki, the renowned sauce/dip eaten with the even more famous Souvlaki, contains olive oil. This is most likely why Greek cuisine is so tasty and nutritious. If you ever visit a Greek kitchen, take advantage of it. It'll almost certainly be brimming with mildly spicy veggies and other spices. You shouldn't be terrified by the prospect of eating their crimson sauces because they omit chile but rather use cinnamon, which enhances the flavour.

Simplicity in Meals

Greek cuisine is simple and elegant, with subtle to robust tastes, smooth to crunchy textures, and an ageless freshness. Preparing and eating Greek food is an exciting excursion into the cradle of civilization and the home of the Gods of Olympus, no matter where you are on the globe. One of the delights we can all share in discovering, tasting, and experiencing Greek cuisine.

Use of Healthy Olive Oil

Greeks are still the top consumers per capita now, but consumption has decreased slightly. Healthy Olive oil has a long history in Greek culture, as it is utilized and continues to be used in practically all Greek table dishes today.

. . .

Unhealthy Influence

Prebiotic fibre supports intestinal health and is found in minimally processed foods, a mainstay in the Greek diet. Throughout the influence of both the eastern and western world in day-to-day lifestyle including food, habits have made Greece sick and unhealthy. Obesity is one of the most prevalent and noticeable side effects of junk food consumption; it is a precursor to difficulties such as diabetes, joint discomfort, and various cardiac diseases. The Mediterranean diet, linked to longer life spans and reduced rates of heart disease and cancer, is currently on the decline in its native region, Greece, where two-thirds of children are overweight, and they are the heaviest smokers in the country. Childhood colds and stomach aches have been replaced by far more dangerous illnesses like diabetes and high blood pressure.

It is the right time for Greeks to go back into their history and learn about the ancient Greeks' healthier and more disciplined eating habits. Limit or eliminate "fast food," which includes items heavy in salt, refined white flour, solid fats or trans fats, and added sweets. Limit or eliminate high-calorie, low-nutrient sodas and other sugar-sweetened beverages. Wholegrain foods such as wholemeal bread, brown rice, and oats can reduce your risk of heart disease and diabetes. They can also aid weight loss by making you feel fuller for longer and reducing the desire for snacking. Modern Greeks should follow the Horta food tradition like their ancestors. Horta is a Greek meal consisting of steamed or cooked leafy green vegetables. After being adequately rinsed, the greens are seasoned with salt and pepper and drizzled with a bit of olive oil and lemon juice.

3
HOW TO IMPLEMENT THE GREEK/MEDITERRANEAN DIET TODAY

There isn't a single Mediterranean diet that everyone follows. People in the Mediterranean have a variety of eating habits, influenced by their geographical, economic, and cultural backgrounds.

What Does It Mean to Follow a Mediterranean Diet? Eating a Mediterranean diet typically means to eat like the people in the Mediterranean region. Freshly produced fruits and vegetables, whole grains, legumes, nutritious fat, and fish from a part of the rich traditional Mediterranean diet. Researchers have always noticed that people in these areas have been incredibly healthy and had a low risk of many diseases (Lăcătușu et al., 2019). The backing of the Mediterranean diet by a ton of scientific evidence proves its benefits, which is why the US News and World Report recently selected the

Mediterranean diet as the number one among over 40 diets they examined.

Let us understand the implementation of the Mediterranean diet in our daily lives with the help of the pyramid. Think of a pyramid divided into four levels. At the lowermost level, you see a lot of fresh fruits and vegetables, whole wheat grains, legumes, lentils, greek yogurt, and all the healthy foods you can think of having today. This level represents the most basic foods an individual must include in their meals. At the second level, Dairy products such as eggs find their place. It suggests that you try to include these every once in a while in your meals. We leave the third level to kinds of seafood and poultry, indicating that you can limit having lean protein to once or twice a week. Finally, the top of the pyramid will find the mention of red meat and sweets advising their consumption only on fewer occasions.

At the basic level, an individual is encouraged to include more fresh fruits and vegetables, whole grains, nuts, and legumes in their daily diet. At the top, the pyramid emphasizes the consumption of lean proteins. A person can consume these from various sources such as fish and poultry. Good fats are paid equal attention in a Mediterranean diet while consuming sweets and red meats on fewer occasions.

. . .

In general,

- One should consume more fresh fruits, leafy vegetables and whole grains every day. One should increase the portion of legumes and nuts in your Mediterranean diet.
- Weekly consumption of lean proteins from fish and poultry is encouraged.
- An individual must altogether limit the consumption of red meats and sweets.
- Eliminating processed foods and too much sugar can help sustain a Mediterranean diet.

Having a busy schedule can make one compromise with this diet. To stick with the Mediterranean diet and achieve one's health goals, one must keep track of what he consumes on the go. Keeping up with the Mediterranean diet is often assumed to be time-consuming, but that's not true! On your busy days, you can choose among plenty of shortcuts at your disposal. Without compromising your nutrition and taste, let us acquaint you with some of the options for your next busy day!

1. A Simple Breakfast Can Save Your Day

That's right, waking up to the thoughts of having a load of work on your shoulders can make you cringe and could affect the rest of your day. To get out of the mess and follow your diet, you can go for nutritious yet time-saving breakfast options like:

- Whole wheat bread with peanut butter is the easiest to follow. It gives energy to your body by providing the right amount of fibre, protein, and fat.
- How about some greek yogurt with fresh berries to start your day?
- You can even consider some cheese with bread.

Mediterranean diets do not include heavy breakfast unless your work demands physical activity.

2. Ready-to-Eat Unprocessed Foods

The Mediterranean diet focuses mainly on including unprocessed foods like fresh fruits and veggies. These are amazing and health-friendly go-to options on a busy day. Greeks have always regularly consumed potatoes, olives, and various seasonal vegetables.

These unprocessed foods can take various forms in a Mediterranean diet. For example, you can include them as a salad to avoid cooking. You can even roast these raw vegetables using extra virgin olive oil, and you are good to go!

3. Frozen Foods Can Save You Time

We all love frozen vegetables. Frozen vegetables like peas can help you save a lot of your time on a busy day. Savouring the taste of greek vegetable casserole Lathera might even lighten your mood. It is easy to prepare and is consumable for over two to three days.

In Greek, Lathera means 'oily,' but the dish we are talking about is not oily. All you need to do is saute onions, add frozen vegetables directly, and some tomato sauce. Put your stove to simmer for some time, and you're all set to savour your Lathera today.

4. How About a Lentil Stew Today?

Everybody loves lentils. They are easy to cook, and there is no need to soak them in water. It takes approximately an hour to make lentil stew. When you have a busy day, you can prepare it in advance. It can also serve as a salad by topping it with tomatoes, olives, etc.

. . .

5. Eggs Can Be Your Whole Meal!

As we know, eggs form an integral part of the Mediterranean or the Greek diet. In Mediterranean regions, eggs form the routine part of the dinner rather than just being limited to breakfast. Hence, you can turn to eggs when you find yourself too tired and confused to prepare your meal. Then, a simple omelet can suffice.

6. Whole Grain Sandwich With Hummus and Vegetables

A wholegrain sandwich with hummus and vegetables will serve as a whole and hearty meal for your Mediterranean diet. Kids everywhere are usually fond of hummus. Hummus is a protein-rich and easily preparable ingredient for the sandwich. A 2016 study reveals that people who consume hummus or chickpeas consume more fibre, protein, unsaturated fats, and more vitamins. All you require are a few loaves of bread, hummus, and fresh vegetables. Its preparation is easy and is tasty yet nutritious.

7. Tzatziki and Melitzanosalata

Tzatziki is a creamy dip prepared by the Greeks. It is made with Greek yogurt, cucumber, and olive oil and is low in calories. It is high in protein and often served as a dip with pita bread. On the days that you feel restless and do not want to cook, you can make this simple dip and have it with pita bread. Melitzanosalata refers to an eggplant salad in Greek. However, Melitzanosalata is a dip. To prepare Melitzanosalata, you need to blend or mash the roasted eggplant with olive oil, garlic, and lemon juice. This antioxidant-rich dish can help you feel full and provide health benefits of its own.

8. Whole Wheat Pasta and Pizza Topped With Feta

You can opt for whole wheat pizza when running on a tight schedule. Greeks tend to eat a lot of pasta and pizza, but they balance them by topping them with fresh vegetables. So going with a whole wheat crust pizza or whole wheat pasta can be your choice of Mediterranean meals on your busy days. If you are fond of cheese, you can top it up with Feta, which is low in fat and calories but tastes delicious.

9. A Healthy Spinach Smoothie Could Be All You Need Today!

How about a glass of a healthy spinach smoothie today? Some spinach, pineapple chunks, diced apples, Greek yogurt, and ice cubes are all you need. Blending them all will make a fresh and green spinach smoothie for you. It is healthy and rich in antioxidants. In addition, spinach provides a generous amount of fibre and vitamins.

10. Souvlaki

Souvlaki is served throughout Greece and is the most popular among the well-known Greek foods. It comprises of small grilled pieces of meat such as pork, chicken, lamb, or beef, which nourish your body with proteins and vitamins. It also leads to increased muscle mass, which is imperative in muscle-building.

11. Avgolemono and Fakes (Greek Style Soups)

Avgolemono is a traditional Greek soup. Its ingredients include lemon, chicken, eggs and rice. Fakes is a soup made with lentils. One can add tomatoes, onions, garlic as per their taste. These soups are an excellent source of protein and fibre. It does not require much time to prepare these greek style soups.

12. A Variety of Snacks (Mezethaki)

On the days that you do not feel the urge to prepare your meals, you open your fridge and put various appetizer-like foods onto your plate. These foods can include basic things like tomatoes, cucumber, olives, feta cheese whole grain pieces of bread, etc. It can satisfy your hunger and, at the same time, fuel your body with energy when you aren't inclined to cook.

13. Spanakorizo

Spanakorizo is a spinach and rice dish prepared with olive oil. You can present it either as a main or a side dish. Again, it is easy to cook. Spinach is among the most healthy vegetables and contains plenty of nutrients. It is rich in vitamin A, Vitamin C, Vitamin K, folic acid, iron, and potassium. Spinach also contains various antioxidants that fight cell damage (Rahal et al., 2014). Likewise, rice is rich in many B-vitamins and minerals like manganese, selenium, and iron. In addition, citric acid and vitamin C contents from the lemon help absorb the contents from Spanakorizo.

14. Mbirgiami (Eggplant and Zuchinni Bake)

This delicious bake includes a variety of vegetables and herbs, such as eggplant, zucchini, parsley, dill and oregano, and is easy to make. It can be served hot or cold, and a great addition to your diet if you want a healthy snack on the go. It also contains many vitamins and nutrients the body needs daily. These low-calorie, low-carb vegetables are an excellent source of vitamin B6, vitamin C and antioxidants. If you sprinkle with feta, you also benefit from the added calcium, which is excellent for bone health. An all-around healthy dish!

15. Nuts and Fruits to Bring Your Hunger Pains to Rest

There are many times during the day when you feel the pains of your hunger. In such situations, one must pick healthier options like having fresh fruit. You can also choose to eat a handful of nuts. An avocado on whole-wheat toast sounds great too! Dried fruits like apricots and figs can also help resolve your mid-day hunger pains. These can also serve as a snack to help you get through your day.

Saying No to Unhealthy Foods

While choosing a Mediterranean diet might help you fulfill all your body goals, you must be watchful of what you consume. The Mediterranean diet was one of the secrets of the longevity of the people who lived on the island Ikaria, Greece. It has attracted the attention of scientists and journalists alike. We know that the Greeks included healthy foods in their everyday life to promote a healthy lifestyle. It enhanced their quality of life. It is well-known that we are what we eat. Therefore, it is of immense importance to cut out things that might be detrimental to our goals when following a Mediterranean diet.

Let us have a look over the foods that we should avoid:

1. Refined grains

Refined grains that include white flour are a big no to your Mediterranean diet. Likewise, followers of the Mediterranean diet should avoid consuming white bread, pizza, and pasta made with white flour.

2. Refined oils

If you are thinking of frying your food in refined soyabean oil, corn oil, vegetable oil, canola oil, or any other hydrogenated oils, you might want to reconsider your options. Looking for healthier options like using extra virgin olive oil can benefit your health.

3. Processed red meats

You should consider cutting the consumption of hot dogs, bacon, lunch meats, and sausage that contain processed red meats. In its report, the World

Health Organization (WHO) mentions that the consumption of red meat is carcinogenic. If on a Mediterranean diet, you can have red meat once in a while. However, you can benefit from cutting its consumption altogether.

4. Processed foods

Cancer is one of the health risks that the Laborer's health and safety fund of North America mentions resulting from consuming processed foods (*The Many Health Risks of Processed Foods*, 2019). Processed foods are high in sugar and sodium. It is for the benefit of the individual that they avoid the consumption of such processed foods. Greek yogurt can replace the urge to have candies and high-sugar desserts for a serving of fresh fruits. It is a healthier option and in line with your Mediterranean diet.

5. Alcohol

Alcohol is the one thing you must avoid while on a Mediterranean diet. It can leave you feeling nauseous. Restlessness, impulsive behaviour, and lack of coordination are some of the side effects of consuming alcohol. It also affects your immune system, making it weaker and leaving you prone to various fatal conditions (Anon, 2021). The Mediterranean diet, however, allows drinking red wine in moderation. Therefore, you can sip on red wine, considering its implications if consumed in excess. Pregnant women should avoid the use of any alcohol.

The Benefits of the Mediterranean Diet

Various organizations around the globe have supported the Mediterranean diet. Let us have a look at their views:

- As per the Mayo Clinic, "The Mediterranean diet is a healthy-eating plan. It's plant-based and incorporates the traditional flavours and cooking methods of the region" (Mayo Clinic Staff, 2019). They say that the Mediterranean diet is a heart-healthy eating plan.
- The American Heart Association says, "This style of eating can play a big role in preventing heart disease and stroke and reducing risk factors such as obesity, diabetes, high cholesterol, and high blood pressure." It emphasizes a diet based on fresh fruits and vegetables, legumes and beans, whole grains, and limited consumption of processed foods (American Heart Association, 2018).

- Harvard mentions, "Research supports the use of the Mediterranean diet as a healthy eating pattern for the prevention of cardiovascular diseases, increasing lifespan, and healthy aging. When used in conjunction with caloric restriction, the diet may also support healthy weight loss" (Boston & Ma 02115 +1495-1000, 2018).

The advantages of a Mediterranean diet have been recognized all over the world. If you choose to shift to a Mediterranean diet and are curious to find out how you can benefit from it, stay with us! We shall guide you through some of its advantages, such as:

- **The Mediterranean diet promotes a healthy heart**

As per a study by the National Institute of Health (NIH), the Mediterranean diet lowers the risk of cardiac arrest and other cardiovascular diseases (Martínez-González et al., 2019). It is a simple phenomenon. Whatever we put into our body, our body reacts accordingly. So, when we consume healthy foods every day, we are less prone to the risk of heart disease.

- **Your blood sugar level stays intact**

Consumption of processed foods and high sodium intake affects our blood sugar level. Therefore, it becomes a challenge to maintain a healthy blood sugar level without a Mediterranean diet. When everything on our diet is in moderation, the possibility of blood sugar levels being stable increases. Also, these diets may help reduce the risk of type-2 diabetes (Martín-Peláez et al., 2020).

- **Improved functioning of the brain**

Many studies have recorded that the Mediterranean diet could help your brain function better. As a result, it could help lower the risk of dementia, cognitive impairment, and Alzheimer's disease (Anon, 2019).

Switching to a Mediterranean diet can positively affect your longevity. As for the curiosity of various scientists and journalists, numerous studies have proved how it makes a person healthier. It promotes a healthy mind; a healthy mind, in turn, will give you a healthy life.

The Greeks in the Mediterranean have always followed a healthy and rich diet. The Mediterranean diet will help give you the tools for a healthy lifestyle and promote your mental well-being. There is no defined Mediterranean diet. This diet mainly consists of plant-based healthy foods and limited consumption of animal-based products once or twice a week.

Its health benefits mainly include helping to stabilize blood sugar levels while promoting a healthy heart rate and facilitating better brain functioning. There is absolutely no doubt why it comes out at a top-ranking among the numerous diets. Best of all, you don't have to stick to any strict diet plan. You can prepare your meals keeping the preference for flavour in your mind. If you dislike a particular thing, such as salmon, you can go for white fish instead.

The Mediterranean diet is a minimal plant-based diet. Therefore, it is not very expensive. You can easily find the ingredients around you to prepare your meals. Also, they are less time-consuming and work fine on your busy days.

Building a Mediterranean diet is simple. The consumption of a plant-based diet keeps you fresh and active throughout the day. It does not promote lethargy, and there is always an option to replace unhealthy foods with healthier ones. Eating a Mediterranean diet is not only healthy but also delicious. If you are thinking of shifting from your regular diet to the Mediterranean, this is the right time!

. . .

What should you invest in on your next grocery run when looking forward to implementing a Mediterranean diet?

When you plan for your entire week and are confused about what to purchase for your upcoming meals, make sure you don't forget to add:

1. Whole wheat grains, oats, barley, whole-wheat pasta, corn, etc.

2. Fresh fruits and vegetables, including broccoli, kale, spinach, onions, cauliflower, etc.

3. The right amount of nuts like cashews, almonds, walnuts, and dried fruits.

4. Legumes, beans, peas, chickpeas and peanuts.

5. Sunflower seeds, pumpkin seeds, flaxseeds and chia seeds.

6. Fish and seafood like salmon, oysters, clams, tuna, trout, etc.

7. Chicken, turkey, duck eggs, and you can also get quail for your meals for the week.

8. Dairy products can include Greek yogurt, Feta cheese, and milk.

9. For healthy fats, make it a point to include extra-virgin olive oil, avocado, and avocado oil.

10. Basil, mint, nutmeg, cinnamon, pepper and ginger.

4

BENEFITS OF A GREEK HOLISTIC DIET/MEDITERRANEAN PLAN

The Mediterranean diet, rooted in the traditional Greek holistic diet, draws inspiration from nations around the Mediterranean Sea such as Greece, Italy, and Spain and is often considered the healthiest eating plan in the world. The Mediterranean diet is moderate and well-balanced, mainly concentrating on regional and seasonal traditional fruits and vegetables, legumes, nuts, seafood, olive oil, and fewer dairy items, aside from a glass of homemade red wine mixed with a bit of water. The Mediterranean diet focuses mainly on healthy dietary principles, such as having a diet rich in fruits and green vegetables. Fruits, vegetables, nuts, herbs, whole grains, olive oil, and legumes comprise most of the Mediterranean diet. These go well together with traditional Greek salad, which consists of tomatoes, cucumbers, red onion, green pepper, olives, and feta cheese.

When it comes to non-vegetarian, lean protein oily fish like salmon and sardines that are high in omega-3 fatty acids are preferred, while eggs and chicken are consumed in smaller amounts every day or a few times a week. Red meat contains a lot of saturated fat, which elevates blood cholesterol and increases the risk of cardiovascular disease. It's obvious why red meats are only served once or twice a month . The Mediterranean diet is more than green vegetables and fruits, seafood, healthy oil, and nutritious foods. Regular physical activity and sharing meals with others are equally important factors. Altogether, they have a powerful impact on the body, helping you stay healthy and strengthening muscles, bones, and joints. This helps improve mood and energy level and enables you to develop an understanding of the delights of consuming nutritious and tasty meals. The Mediterranean dietary principles and lifestyle can help people combat chronic disease, lower their risk of cardiovascular disease, and live a longer, healthier life.

Health Benefits **of a Mediterranean Diet Plan**

Since ancient times, the Mediterranean diet has been known for its dietary disciplines, selection of highly nutritious foods, and well-combined healthy foods. These foods are abundant in nutrients that have apparent positive effects on the heart, brain, and whole body, leading to a long and healthy life. Here are some health benefits of the Greek diet plan that you need to know:

1. Reduced risk of Heart Disease and Stroke

A Mediterranean diet restricts your consumption of refined bread, processed foods, and red meat. In addition, it reduces the risk of cardiovascular disease by lowering saturated fat consumption and adopting a calorie-unrestricted diet with extra-virgin olive oil or almond oil.

Including fish high in omega-3 fatty acids in the diet improves the heart by promoting healthy levels of good HDL cholesterol. Omega-3 fatty acids benefit persons with high blood pressure and heart disease. It reduces the development of inflammatory substances in the body. No wonder why Greeks made fish as a primary non-vegetarean meal over red meat in their diet.

The majority of Greeks prefer wine over other alcoholic beverages. Wine is mixed with one-third of water to avoid getting inebriated. High in natural polyphenols, such as those found in grapes used to make red wine, reduce the risk of Ischemic heart problems. The Mediterranean diet is one of the most well-studied nutritional patterns regarding cardiovascular disease risk and other health outcomes. It has helped prevent overall and particular forms of heart disease, perhaps to a moderate-high degree.

2. Improves Brain Health

A Mediterranean balanced diet style of eating lowers inflammation in the body, defends against many types of cell damage, lowers blood pressure, and helps maintain healthy cholesterol levels. In addition, according to a study by the American Academy of Neurology, over three years, individuals who followed the Mediterranean diet more closely kept larger brain volume than those who did not (Anon, 2019).

This study looked at 967 Scottish adults in their 70s who had never experienced dementia. Out of 562 participants, 401 underwent two MRI brain scans within three years. It was observed that people who did not follow the Mediterranean diet adequately had a higher loss of total brain value than those who did. The difference in total brain volume between the two groups of participants was 0.5 percent. The study also revealed that eating habits and food might preserve the brain in the long run. Other studies are also being conducted. A Greek diet may help in the prevention of Alzheimer's disease. According to the American Academy of Neurology Research, eating a diet rich in unsaturated fats, seafood, fruits, and vegetables, while avoiding dairy and red meat might help clear the brain from protein accumulation that causes memory loss and dementia. They found that participants who followed the Mediterranean diet regularly on a long-term basis had less brain volume shrinkage and protein indicators linked to Alzheimer's disease (Alzheimer's Association, 2021).

3. Balanced Body Weight and Fit Life

Unlike in Western nations, where meat consumption is rampant and has become a daily dish on the plate, the Mediterranean diet is more vegetarian and has managed to limit its meat. Fat is prominent, mainly unsaturated fat in red meat and poultry. Eating a lot of saturated fat increases your risk of coronary heart disease as it raises cholesterol in the blood. Therefore, it's more challenging to maintain healthy body weight when consuming meat. Following healthy seafood and limiting consumption of chicken, beef, or bacon is undoubtedly a healthy idea, and Greeks have been doing it for a long time.

Plant-based foods, primarily vegetables and fruits, make up a large percentage of the Mediterranean diet. Vegetarian foods are naturally low in fat and calories and high in dietary fibre. Vegetables come in a wide range, which allows for a lot of experimentation in the kitchen. Seasonal vegetables are a good source of various beneficial nutrients found in cabbage, turnips, kale, mandarins, lemons, asparagus, rhubarb, fennel, green leafy vegetables, and artichokes. These seasonal fruits and vegetables are a good source of fibre and nutrients, including essential minerals, antioxidants, and vitamins, which may promote your body, optimize your metabolism, and burn belly fat. Incorporating these foods into your diet may assist you in maintaining a healthy weight.

4. Beneficial to Diabetics

People with type 2 diabetes may benefit more from a Mediterranean-style diet than a typical low-fat diet to keep their illness under control without medicines. Reduced meat consumption, moderate wine intake, reasonably less dairy consumption, easily digested whole grain bread, as well as other cereals and legumes as dietary staples, traditional salad, nuts and seeds, fruit desserts, pressed extra-virgin olive oil, and regular physical activity all contribute to maintaining a healthy weight and lifestyle. The Mediterranean diet's positive impact on blood glucose levels is likely owing to the diet's emphasis on complex carbohydrates, which take longer to digest and do not increase blood sugar levels. In addition, healthy choices result in a diet high in monounsaturated fat and fibre, both of which can decrease cholesterol and blood sugar in people with diabetes.

5. Natural and Unprocessed

Greek cuisine generally uses more 'whole' and 'raw' ingredients in its meals, which means they are frequently closer to nature and less processed. Greek cuisine has low fructose corn syrup, genetically modified organisms (GMOs), or other artificial additives. It also utilizes less red meat and employs more plant-based foods, wild-caught seafood, and legumes. When combined with olive oil, these nutritional elements significantly improve the health benefits.

6. May help in the Prevention of Cancer

The Mediterranean diet has long been associated with a reduced risk of cancer because Lactobacillus bacteria from the mammary gland are more prevalent in the Mediterranean diet. Breast cancer development has been proven to be slowed by these bacteria. In addition, malignant breast tumours have a lower abundance of Lactobacillus than noncancerous breast tumours.

Those who eat a Mediterranean diet have higher bile acid metabolites, lowering their risk of breast cancer. This is because a microbiota exists in the breast glands. It, too, maybe influenced by nutrition, much like the gut microbiota. The term' microbiome' refers to a collection of living organisms that inhabit our bodies, such as bacteria and fungus. The health of this ecosystem is critical. Fish, olive oil, vegetables, whole grains, nuts, and legumes are abundant in a typical Mediterranean diet. Since the diet is low in red meat, dairy, and moderate alcohol intake, it can lower cancer risk and help them live longer.

7. Tackling With Depression and Anxiety

Cooking with olive oil, a good source of monounsaturated fat, is common in Mediterranean-style diets. Mediterranean diets are thought to lower cardiovascular risk, delay bone loss in osteoporosis, encourage anti-cancer pathways, and enhance brain health, as well as being linked to a lower incidence of depression, according to "Healthy Brain." Dietary changes are a viable treatment for depression that has few adverse effects, slows illness development, and is a cost-effective approach adopted worldwide. According to current research, more objective metrics are needed to characterize the Mediterranean diet, which underscores the necessity for longitudinal investigations and clinical trials in the future. Methodological differences in Mediterranean diets hampered comparisons but resolved by defining inclusion criteria and compressive data analysis. Dietary changes are a viable therapy for depression with few adverse effects and slow illness development.

Scientific Benefits of Healthy Elements of the Mediterranean Diet:

Vegetables and Herbs

Leafy greens have been an integral part of the daily diet since prehistoric times. They should be included in any healthy diet plan because they are high in various vitamins and minerals. In addition, green vegetables are high in fibre and low in fat and sugar, which makes them perfect for a weight-loss diet. They also safeguard your body by boosting immunity, reducing the aging process, and avoiding heart disease, increased blood pressure, and cancer.

Fresh green vegetables and herbs are abundant in antioxidants and anti-inflammatory chemicals. In traditional Greek cuisine, they contribute considerably to the overall dietary intake of flavonols and flavones. Each region of the Mediterranean has its distinct flavour profile, yet herbs and spices are ubiquitous in Mediterranean cooking. To boost antioxidant capability, do like the Greeks do and add fresh herbs to salads. Many traditional plants in North America grow wild along Mediterranean highways.

Wine

The great taste of red wine and the various circumstances that enable one to enjoy it are undeniable. However, what may come as a surprise is that its antioxidant concentration has been linked to multiple health benefits, ranging from cancer prevention to mental health and longer life expectancy. Alcohol intake is popular in the traditional Mediterranean diet but typically in moderation and, as a rule, at meals. In the spirit of the old Greek word symposium—wine, particularly red wine, is high in antioxidant polyphenols and flavonoid resveratrol, which may help raise HDL cholesterol while lowering LDL cholesterol. Acquiring antioxidants through food is likely to be healthier than drinking wine. Moderate red wine consumption is linked to lower cancer risk or better results.

Whole Grain Wheat

Wheat is the Mediterranean's most important crop. Farro/emmer (Triticum dicoccum), ancient wheat with increased appeal in Italy and the United

States, is one traditional grain. Bulgur is formed from steamed, dried, and cracked whole wheat berries and used in pilafs, tabbouleh, and kibbe, a classic Lebanese meal of minced meat with bulgur and spices. For bulgur, coarse is best for pilafs, the medium is best for tabbouleh and other salads, and fine is best for kibbe.

Unrefined wheat and barley flour are frequently used in bread. The classic Mediterranean wheat, durum, has a creamy yellow hue from natural carotenoids and is used for bread, couscous, and Italian pasta. Wheat was initially processed with millstones, giving a fibre-rich whole-wheat flour with a lower glycemic index than today's modern refined flours. It was additionally leavened using a sourdough starter, which lowered the glycemic index of the wheat flour during fermentation. If you're trying to lose weight, whole wheat bread is the way to go because it's high in fibre. You won't have any trouble incorporating whole wheat bread into your diet because bread is already versatile. In addition, whole wheat bread is high in vitamins and minerals, which helps you stay energized all day. These nutrients can help you feel more energized and possibly accelerate your metabolism.

OLIVE OIL

Oil is the common denominator in the many

dietary patterns that make up the general Mediterranean diet. Tocopherols, carotenoids, and polyphenols are abundant in extra-virgin olive oil, providing antioxidant and anti-inflammatory qualities. Olive oil is essential in promoting a high vegetable- and legume-consumption diet. Olive oil is also used in baking and cooking. Contrary to popular assumptions because of its decreased free fatty acid content, high-quality extra-virgin olive oil has a high smoke point.

This liquid gold is hailed for nothing as a vital element of one of the primary pillars of a Mediterranean diet, possibly the world's healthiest diet. Olive oil is more beneficial than other oils due to its high nutritional content and has various health advantages. Antioxidants are known to protect cells from cellular damage caused by free radicals created by the body during activities such as metabolism. Oxidative stress caused by a build-up of free radicals in the body can cause cell damage and is thought to play a role in developing illnesses like cancer. Using olive oil for cooking and eating can lower the incidence of breast cancer and prevent colorectal cancer. Heart disease, type 2 diabetes, obesity, arthritis, cancer, and other disorders is caused by chronic inflammation. Olive oil antioxidants, particularly oleocanthal, operate similarly to anti-inflammatory medicines to reduce inflammation.

. . .

Greek Feta and Yogurt

Greek yogurt and Feta are excellent protein, fat, and carbohydrates sources and are high in many nutrients. Feta is available in a variety of fat levels, including total fat, reduced fat, and fat-free, as well as flavoured and unflavored variants, with no additions or preservatives allowed. When purchasing Feta, check for a PDO stamp or text indicating that it is PDO authorized, as well as a clear label stating that it is" Greek feta" rather than feta-style cheese. Like all other dairy products, Feta is high in calcium, necessary for nerve and muscle function and strong, healthy teeth and bones. A serving of cheese provides a valuable contribution to your daily calcium requirements, which is vital at all stages of life. In addition, Feta is a helpful nutritional addition due to its high-protein content, especially for lacto-vegetarians.

Because Feta and yogurt are fermented, they are high in probiotics. They also contribute protein to a predominantly plant-based diet. Feta cheese is commonly served with stews and the traditional Greek salad. Goat's milk or sheep's milk make authentic Greek Feta. The Greeks most likely introduced yogurt, and it is now more widely used throughout the eastern Mediterranean. Greek yogurt with honey is a popular breakfast option. Protein is vital for optimal health since it is the building block of muscle, skin, and blood, and we require enough quantities in our meals for cells and tissues to grow, expand, and heal.

Lemon

Acidic meals reduce stomach emptying, which lowers glycemic response. Lemon peels' acidity and high flavonoid content may assist in managing or preventing diabetes by lowering blood glucose levels. Lemons and oranges are native to the Far East, and they were first introduced to the Mediterranean by Arabs. Squeezing lemons over salads, seafood, soups, and beans, as well as into drinking water, is a widespread Mediterranean practice that lowers the glycemic load of the entire meal.

Lemons include vitamins, fibre, and plant chemicals that can benefit one's health. The pulp, rind, and juice are high in vitamins that boost immunity and lower illness risk. Lemon's soluble dietary fibre promotes digestive health. Lemons and other citrus fruits are high in vitamin C, an effective antioxidant protecting cells from free radical damage. You've undoubtedly heard that vitamin C can help some people avoid or shorten the length of a cold, but Research is mixed. Vitamin C has been shown to lower blood pressure and reduce your risk of cardiovascular disease and stroke.

. . .

Garlic

Garlic is a critical element in many Mediterranean cuisines; the garlic used differs by region. Tzatziki is a famous Eastern Mediterranean sauce made with yogurt, garlic, cucumbers, olive oil, red wine vinegar, and salt. Another typical dish is Aioli, which combines garlic, eggs, and olive oil. Garlic's sulphur components are responsible for its pungent odour as well as the majority of its health advantages, including anticancer, antioxidant, and anti-inflammatory properties. When added to one's diet, raw garlic can help with digestive disorders. It is beneficial to the intestines and aids in the relief of inflammation. In addition, eating raw garlic can help you get rid of intestinal worms. It destroys bad bacteria while conserving helpful bacteria in the stomach, which is positive.

A chemical found in garlic called Allicin prevents LDL (bad cholesterol) from oxidizing. It aids in the reduction of cholesterol and the promotion of heart health. Garlic consumption reduces the occurrence of blood clots, which helps to prevent thromboembolism. Garlic also decreases blood pressure, making it beneficial to hypertensive people. Many health practitioners believe raw garlic can ward off a cough and cold illness. The most significant benefit comes from eating two smashed cloves of garlic on an empty stomach. Garlic cloves strung around the necks of children and newborns are said to reduce congestion problems.

Seafood and Omega-3 Fatty Acids

In modern Greek cuisine, meat consumption has decreased significantly. Greeks have reduced their meat and poultry consumption due to the adverse effects on their bodies and minds. Instead, they've shifted to a more nutritious and delectable sea-based choice such as sardines, salmon, squid, octopus, and other lean protein sources. In Greece, sardines and salmon are two of the most popular fish. These tiny, fatty fish are not only delicious, but they are also one of the healthiest meals available. Sardines are abundant in protein and omega-3 fatty acids, reducing the risk of heart disease. Salmon are abundant in vitamin D, potassium, and omega-3 fatty acids and contain numerous vitamins and minerals, including calcium and vitamin D for healthy bones. Omega-3 fatty acids are abundant in this fish. Omega-3 fatty acids can help your heart and circulatory system. Omega-3 fatty acids also assist in preventing blood platelets from clumping together, lowering the risk of blood clots. Slowing the formation of triglycerides in the liver reduces triglyceride levels. Triglyceride levels in the blood are linked to an increased risk of heart disease.

Long-term sustainable dietary adjustments are a

requirement of the Mediterranean diet. In general, a diet rich in natural foods, such as an abundance of vegetables, whole grains, and nutritious fats, should be the goal. Anyone who doesn't feel satisfied with their diet should consult a dietician. They might suggest more or different foods to aid with satiety. Regularly following a Greek diet might be one of the healthiest decisions you ever undertake. It's also an excellent diet for losing weight safely and healthily.

5
GREEK DIET AND ITS BENEFITS TO VARIOUS BODY SYSTEMS

The Greek diet is much more than just a healthy, nutritious diet for the body and mind. The Greek diet focuses on what is simply good for you while eliminating what isn't suitable for your body. The advantages of the Greek diet plan are not just limited to the nutritional values it provides; it also has significant benefits to the human body's systems. You don't have to fly to Greece to follow the Greek diet; it can be achieved by keeping a healthy balance of what to eat and what not to eat, regular physical activity, and companionship. There's a reason it's regarded as the greatest eating plan on the planet. So rather than fried chicken, try fish. Instead of a white flour roll, use brown rice. Take a handful of almonds rather than chips. Instead of butter, use olive oil—also, plenty of fruits and veggies.

Greek food is both healthy and delicious, and it's high in antioxidants, fibre, good fats, minerals, and vitamins, all of which have been linked to improved health. It may provide your body with adequate nutrition and put you in a great spot to battle chronic illness by boosting Greek staples like fruits, vegetables, herbs, olive oil, seafood, and lean meats in your diet. According to some studies, eating a Greek diet might be one of the healthiest moves you ever make. Heart disease, cancer, high blood pressure, diabetes, digestive and intestinal tract, stress, and Alzheimer's disease can all be reduced by eating a traditional Greek diet. It's also an excellent diet for losing weight safely and healthily. A switch to a Greek diet may be just what you need to improve various aspects of your health, physique, or life.

HEALTH BENEFITS of Greek Diets for Various Bodily Systems:

PREVENTS GASTROINTESTINAL PROBLEMS

The Greek Diet is a diverse combination of dietary factors practiced by people living in Mediterranean regions. It includes a high intake of olive oil, fibre-rich meals, milk or dairy products, and a reduced intake of red meat and meat-based items. Since ancient times, the Mediterranean coast has followed an essential diet that may offer long-term health secrets. However, maintaining gut homeostasis requires a balanced diet as well.

Gastrointestinal disorders have become a common yet serious problem these days. Issues related to the intestinal tract can be life-threatening in some cases. These unfavourable consequences are caused by the by-products of fatty acid breakdown in the gastrointestinal system and throughout the body. The microbiomes in our gastrointestinal system create chemical signals and metabolites as they process and digest the foods we eat, which can cause the body to react in undesired ways, such as increasing inflammation, changing immunity, and modifying metabolism. Functional gastrointestinal disorders (FGIDs), like functional dyspepsia (FD) or irritable bowel syndrome (IBS), can be triggered by specific dietary regimes or even certain meals (IBS). Food impacts on microbiota composition and luminal distension are associated with gas generation from bacterial fermentation. Immediate effects of specific nutrients on GI sensitivity and motility are all examples of FGIDs. The Greek diet may also help with functional gastrointestinal issues.

A diet low in red meat and poultry and high in fruits, vegetables, and healthy fats, such as the Greek diet, has been shown in several studies to reduce inflammation and support a healthy digestive system. In addition, microbes in the gastrointestinal system are essential for optimal digestion, and a diet high in plant-based foods may help.

GREEK DIET PLAN **Aids for Digestive Disorders**

In today's frantic modern age, the new generation has discovered shortcuts to eating, just as they have found shortcuts to other things; nevertheless, this shortcut is also a shortcut to inviting diseases into their lives and, more specifically, into their stomach. Junk food has embraced the new generation. This practice has become common in Western countries. It has not spared the nations around the Mediterranean Sea, and its adverse effects are apparent. Yet, most Greeks still adhere to the traditional Greek dietary system, which shields them from the harmful effects of junk food and the substances it contains (junk food is often highly saturated in fat).

Junk food ingredients can harm bodily systems, especially the digestive system. Fast food can contain various elements that are incompatible with a healthy diet. Many quick meals are high in carbs, which our digestive system struggles to digest. These carbohydrates convert down into glucose, or sugar, which raises your blood sugar. Long-term use of fast food can result in insulin resistance, type 2 diabetes, and weight gain. From high blood pressure and cholesterol to blood sugar surges and weight gain, it's evident that fast food typically lacks the nutrients the body needs while also introducing excessive amounts of a diet we don't require. Sugar and fat levels are high. Extra (empty) calories result from the addition of sugar. It's also a risk to your cardiovascular system, leading to heart disease. Foods heavy in fat, particularly trans-fat, can raise bad cholesterol and reduce good cholesterol.

The unique feature of the Greek diet that makes it so beneficial for stomach problems is that it often eliminates meats that are typically high in fat, which makes them hard to digest. The unique feature of the Greek diet that makes it so beneficial is the selection of healthy, green leafy vegetables and fruits, which are easy to digest and incorporate into one's nutritious diet. Inclination towards season fruits and vegetables are appropriate for that geographical location and meet the body's demands. More accessible proteins, such as fish and lentils, will aid digestion and leave you feeling full and less bloated after each meal. Vegetarian meals are inherently low in fat, calories, and nutritional fibre.

The Greek diet shows how to avoid stomach disorders by eliminating a few eatables from your kitchen, unlike in Western and Asian nations where milk and other dairy products are an integral part of the diet. Dairy products such as high-fat milk, butter, and cheese can't seem to find any particular place in Greek households, maybe because they were never given a high priority. Milk's adverse effects were known to the ancient Greeks.

Dairy is one food type that might be difficult to digest due to lactose, a sugar present in milk, and other dairy products. Even if dairy does not make you sick, you may be lactose intolerant. Gas and bloating occur when lactose isn't absorbed correctly, as it occurs in those with lactose intolerance. Other digestive disorders such as bloating, cramps, or diarrhea may occur. When lactose is ingested in excess, it reaches the large intestine, leading to diarrhea. Lactose passes through your digestive tract and is broken down by gut bacteria through a fermentation process if you can't break it down readily. Gassiness and other digestive issues linked with lactose intolerance are unwanted consequences of this approach. If you have digestive issues, yogurt and hard cheeses may be good to consume because they don't contain lactose, or you can try lactose-free milk.

Soothes Inflammation and Digestive Tract Problems

The Greek diet relies heavily on olive oil. Olive oil is often regarded as the Mediterranean diet's signature food ingredient. Many of the health advantages of this diet can be linked to olive oil's beneficial characteristics. More significant consumption of plant-based oils, such as olive oil, is beneficial for an inflamed digestive tract. Inflammation can be reduced, and a healthy digestive system can be promoted by following a Greek diet. Microbes in the gastrointestinal system are essential for optimal digestion, and foods high in plant-based consumption may help.

The function of your big and small intestines is to digest food and transport nutrients throughout your body. Extra-virgin olive oil can promote adequate bile drainage and thorough gallbladder emptying. This is one of the benefits of extra-virgin olive oil on the hepato-biliary system or a healthy digestive system. Another consequence is that it promotes gallbladder contractions, which is particularly beneficial in treating and preventing bile duct problems. In addition, it raises the quantity of cholesterol secreted by the liver and enhances the creation of bile salts in the liver. Inflammation can be reduced, and a healthy digestive system can be promoted by following a Greek diet. Diets high in fibre, such as whole grains, legumes, nuts, seeds, fruits, and green leafy vegetables, are part of the Greek diet. The fibre in these meals nourishes gut bacteria, aiding regularity and promoting a healthy gut environment. Inflammation can be reduced, and a healthy digestive system can be promoted by following a Greek diet.

. . .

Promotes Good Gut Bacteria

A Greek diet has been shown to impact the microbiome ecosystem network positively. Obesity is a serious health concern among metabolic illnesses, and a Greek Dietary program may help halt its progression. Microbes in the gastrointestinal tract are essential for good digestion and may benefit from a diet rich in plant-based foods. Greek diet choices appear to influence gut microbiota and shape its composition considerably. High-fat diets alter the gut microbiota unfavourably, leading to dysbiosis, whereas plant-based diets have a favourable impact. As a result, the gut microbiota may provide information about one's eating patterns and reflect whether or not one eats a healthy diet. The gut microbiota is implicated in various host metabolic pathways and has a critical role in immunological and metabolic homeostasis, which is more than an assumption.

It can aid in the digestion of nutrients that would otherwise be inaccessible to the human body and participate in the metabolism of carbohydrates, resulting in the production of short-chain fatty acids like omega-3. Butyrate, acetate, and propionate are all vital energy sources for the host. Furthermore, it is involved in vitamin production, lipolysis, and the formation of the intestinal mucosa. Finally, creating antimicrobial chemicals and limiting their colonization protects its host from harmful germs.

Numerous studies have shown that following the Greek diet has a significant influence on the makeup of gut bacteria. Probiotics are "good bacteria," naturally found. It promotes well-being and is related to longevity with a low prevalence of chronic diseases.

LOWERS Your Cardiovascular Risk

A healthy heart demands a balanced diet, an organized everyday routine, and avoiding junk foods, refined bread, processed foods, dairy, poultry, and red meat. Reduce saturated fat consumption by using extra-virgin olive oil or almond oil in a calorie-unrestricted diet. So, this is what a traditional Greek diet looks like. A Greek diet can help to lower the risk of cardiovascular disease.

The Greek diet has been associated with a reduced risk of diabetes and dementia. It's well-known for its heart-health benefits: Persons who follow a Greek diet over time have a much lower cardiovascular risk than non-followers. However, a recent study reveals that following a Mediterranean diet can reduce cardiovascular risk by up to 30% in patients following a proper diet regularly. Some other benefits of a healthy diet may outweigh the benefits of statins, one of the most often prescribed cardiac medications.

Primed trial (Prevention Con Dieta Mediterranean) shows that a Greek diet rich in olive oil and almonds lowers the risk of cardiovascular disease compared to a low-fat diet advised by the Greek diet plan. The research involved 7,447 people who were free of cardiac disease but had a high risk of cardiovascular disease. The participants were divided into three groups and given three diet plans: one with extra-virgin oil, one with minimal fat, and one with nuts. None of the diets included calorie restriction and increased physical activity (Harvard School of Public Health, 2018). The effects of a Greek diet on the risk of cardiovascular disease were investigated in this study. In addition, this research compared the impact of a Greek diet on individuals over five years to those who did not eat a Greek diet. The study's goal was to see how a Greek diet affected people's health.

Compared to a low-fat diet, the Greek diet dramatically lowered the risk of heart attack, stroke, and heart-related mortality. However, researchers recognized shortcomings in the study's methodology and were forced to retract the conclusions. The most serious flaw was that not all subjects were randomly assigned to their diet, which impacted the outcomes. Nevertheless, the researchers could reanalyze the data and resolve the problem. Compared to a low-fat diet, the Mediterranean diet plan, plus olive oil or almonds, lowered the risk of cardiac events by around 30% for people with high blood pressure, cholesterol issues, or diabetes. In addition, the Greek diet worked better for obesity than the control diet. Researchers say that when it comes to a healthy diet, the Greek Diet is no less than a proper planned diet in its way (Harvard School of Public Health, 2018).

Reduced **Risk of Coronary Artery Disease**

The risk of coronary artery disease is highly adversely associated with the traditional Greek diet. As a result, Greek men live longer than males from other European nations or North America. In addition, several aspects of the traditional Greek diet may play a role in preventing coronary heart disease from developing. They include high consumption of olive oil, which significantly increases the ratio of heart problems, regular consumption of fibre-rich legumes and vegetables. These meals cooked with olive oil, higher consumption of fruits and vegetables, and moderate wine consumption intensifies heart problems without huge intoxication risks.

Diets rich in fruits, vegetables, legumes, and whole grains, as well as fish, nuts, and low-fat dairy products, provide health advantages. These nutritional traits are reflected in the traditional Greek diet, in which olive oil is the primary source of fat. A considerable amount of data has identified links between the Greek diet and all-cause mortality, coronary heart disease, and several forms of cancer in the last few decades. In addition, the findings of research linked the Greek diet to a decreased incidence of coronary heart disease (American Heart Association, 2018b).

Diet's Feature for a Happy Heart

Much of the significant dietary modifications that can assist in maintaining your heart health are naturally included in the typical Mediterranean diet. So, instead of relying on starchy carbs like wholegrain bread and spaghetti, consider including more fruits, vegetables, and salads, including tomatoes, into your diet. If you want to eat better for your heart, the Greek diet is a deliciously healthy choice. According to studies, eating a Greek diet with olive oil or almonds can help lower the risk of heart attack and stroke when contrasted to a low-fat diet. This is due to the emphasis on healthy fats, antioxidants, and high-potassium meals such as fruits and vegetables (Gunnars, 2017).

The Greek diet's main features are limited consumption of poultry and meat products, with very little red meat (lamb, beef, pork) being only eaten on special occasions, very little or no consumption of cured foods, butter, ice creams, or other dairy products. At the same time, cheese and yogurt were consumed in moderate amounts due to the high intake of fresh, seasonal, locally grown vegetables, fruits, nuts, legumes, and grains, rich in nutrients and fibre. Fish is high in good fatty acids, and shellfish are a source of protein. The Greek diet appears to be an optimal nutritional model for cardiovascular health. It is high in plant-based foods, low in saturated fat, meats, and dairy products, and high in monounsaturated fat from olive oil.

Helps **Alleviate Chronic Stress**

Homo sapiens' ancestors separated from the ancestors of other primates at different periods, which means we're connected to certain monkeys closely and distantly to others. Humans and monkeys are both basic creatures with a lot in common. Monkeys are incredibly clever and possess a profound sense of emotion, including stress.

Research on middle-aged monkeys was done to find the effects of a Greek diet on stress and anxiety in primates. The monkeys on the Greek diet were shown to be more robust than those fed a western diet heavy in protein, saturated fat, salt, and sugar. It has a similar effect on humans, and the Greek diet is beneficial in reducing tension and anxiety (Harvard School of Public Health, 2018).

Chronic stress is a long-term feeling of anxiety that, if left untreated, can harm health. It can be spurred on by regular family and job demands, as well as traumatic events. Stress responses are all too common due to our contemporary lifestyle and foods. Yes, your food may affect your mood and stress level. People are driven to overeat by stress, the chemicals it releases, and the impact of high-fat, sugary "delicious dessert." When it comes to diet, stress can suppress appetite in the near term. The neurological system instructs the adrenal glands, located on top of the kidneys, to release the hormone epinephrine (also known as adrenaline). Epinephrine aids in the activation of the body's battle or run response, a heightened physiological state that momentarily halts appetite.

When you stress, adrenal glands release cortisol, also known as the stress hormone. Cortisol is healthy for a short period as a protective mechanism. However, too much cortisol creates stress in your body in the long term, leading to more inflammation and raising the pulse rate. Meanwhile, it seems to have the complete opposite effect in the short term. Focusing on an anti-inflammatory diet is the greatest strategy to reduce cortisol levels in the body. When you're anxious, you should eat a variety of foods (fish, poultry, fruits, vegetables, whole grains, and healthy fats) from the Greek diet. These foods lower cortisol levels by reducing inflammation in the body—whole grains, which are high in vitamin B and vitamin B-12, aid in regulating Cortisol metabolism.

Olive oil is highly crucial in the Greek diet for

various reasons. Olive oil is high in omega-3 fatty acids, which have been shown to decrease inflammation. Sardines, salmon, and tuna fish, likewise strong in omega-3 fatty acids, are popular among Greek adults and may have similar effects. Magnesium-rich foods including avocados, bananas, spinach, broccoli, and others lower stress hormone, metabolism, and inflammation, which soothes the body.

Greeks do not prefer animal protein such as beef, pig, poultry, etc., except in the form of fish. However, eating meat high in protein and lentils, almonds, and peanuts provides a decent source of protein that helps maintain a healthy blood sugar level, which can help reduce stress levels. The Greek diet excludes dairy products, but yogurt is everyone's favourite because of its gut-friendly nature, low cholesterol, and balanced sugar level, which refreshes the body and mind. Hard beverages can elevate cortisol levels, but grape wine is mild in alcoholic qualities and usually blended with water to avoid being inebriated.

The Benefits of a Greek Diet on the Immune System:

The importance of a Greek-style diet rich in plant foods that provide vitamins, minerals, polyphenols, and prebiotic fibre cannot be understated. Nutrients found in fruits and vegetables, such as beta-carotene, vitamin C, and vitamin E, can help the immune system work better. In addition, antioxidants are abundant in many vegetables, fruits, and other plant-based diets, and they aid in minimizing oxidative stress and help your immune system. This will assist the body in fighting infections and reduce chronic systemic inflammation, which is linked to non-communicable illnesses. Many non-communicable chronic diseases (cardiovascular disease, rheumatoid arthritis, type 2 diabetes) have chronic systemic inflammation as a critical underlying feature. Eating patterns such as the Mediterranean diet have been well researched and known for reducing the risk of these diseases, with some research finding positive aspects at the advantages of daily physical activity (Team, 2020).

Many vitamins and minerals are essential for our immune system, including vitamin A, C, and E, rich in the Mediterranean diet's fresh fruits and vegetables. In addition, fresh fruit is well-known for being an excellent source of vitamin C and is used freely in the preparation of various plant foods such as vegetables, salads, legumes, and grains. These foods provide nutrients, boost nutrient absorption and, most significantly, enhance flavour. After all, the Mediterranean Diet's taste makes it so tempting and long-term viable.

Our body's equilibrium and health regulation require a proper interplay between our immune system and gut bacteria. Many features of the Greek diet are beneficial to our digestive health. A diet rich in fruits and vegetables, such as the Mediterranean diet, is high in antioxidants, particularly polyphenols, a class of chemicals that exhibit antioxidant activity. Polyphenols are recognized to have a crucial function in our immune system by reducing inflammation. Fruits, veggies, herbs, spices, extra virgin olive oil, cereals, tea, nuts, seeds, certain grains, legumes, and wine contain dietary phenols. These items are commonly found in the Greek diet high in phenolic compounds.

The importance of good gut flora for a robust immune system cannot be overstated. When polyphenols and other elements of plant food termed prebiotic fibre are digested, they function as food for gut bacteria. A prebiotic is a fibre that must go undigested through the gastrointestinal tract to increase the growth and activity of certain' good' bacteria in the digestive tract.

Making yogurt a part of your healthy diet is a good idea. Yogurt is high in vitamins and protein, but it also contains lactobacillus, a probiotic (good bacteria) that aids in the battle against infection and boosts your immune system.

Eating Together and Companionship

Food played an important role in the Ancient Greeks' efforts to develop a civilized lifestyle that differentiated them from barbarians. Animals and so-called barbarians also ate together, but what made a meal' social' was explicit norms (for example, the appropriate manner of pouring wine) and sociability (eating and drinking with good company). To the Greeks, eating is about finding happiness and living in the moment, easily converting a simple family supper into an all-night affair. Eating with others is beneficial to one's physical and mental well-being. One characteristic that distinguishes Greek families from other cultures is that they always cook together.

Meals prepared and consumed in the company regularly are more nutritional and healthier. According to studies, people who eat meals socially consume more fruits and vegetables, dairy, and fibre than those who eat alone (Anon, 2021a). It makes little difference whether the day's main meal is consumed in the afternoon, as it is in much of Greece, or the evening, as has been increasingly usual in recent years as Greeks have adhered to traditional business hours. Preparing dinner together is part of the joy of sharing a meal. Even though this is done worldwide, the Greeks manage to make it a communal affair.

Eating is a particularly social affair in contemporary Greece. While eating supper or lunch, it is common for individuals to unwind and engage in lively debates on topics ranging from politics to relationships. Anorexia, alcoholism, aggressive behaviour, sadness, and suicidal thoughts under stress and depression in teens can all be avoided by having regular family dinners. Aside from overall fitness and health, social engagement table manners and conversations about current events can help children become better at communicating and interacting. It's a way of life that involves food sharing with family and friends, nutrition, physical activity, and company. One of its distinguishing features is the emphasis on family dinners, which include all family members from all generations sitting together and eating a wholesome diet.

6

OLIVE OIL AND ITS ANCIENT GREEK HISTORY

Olives are indisputably the healthiest of fruits. You can find mention of olives in various religious texts and by numerous philosophers and poets. The origination of olive trees dates back thousands of years. They have been a topic of discussion among many writers across the globe. It is a native of the Mediterranean region, specifically of present-day Turkey. Olives have provided nutrition to the Mediterranean people for ages. In our modern world, the use of olives is not limited to the Mediterranean region but spreads across the globe. Olives offers food, medicinal potions, and nourishing oils. Olive trees are a legend in themselves. They can stand tall for thousands of years and are known for their strength and longevity. Olives have always brought about vitality and good health. Ancient Greeks used olives for cooking, making perfumes, soaps, and ointments. They considered it a fountain of wealth, liquid gold, and the great healer.

Mediterranean people were aware of the potential health benefits of the olives. Therefore, they would extract oils from the olive and use them in cooking. Olive oil is the basis of the Greek Mediterranean diet. Let us understand the origin and history of Greek olive oil.

The Origin and History of Greek Olive Oil

Scientists say that the olive tree sprung up in the Mediterranean region for the first time. The first-ever cultivation of olives began in Crete in about 3,500 BC. During that time, olive trees looked somewhat different. They were wilder, more intense, and played a significant role in maintaining their economy. The export of olive oil started from Crete to various regions in Greece, North Africa, and Asia. The production of olive trees and oil then passed to mainland Greece, where Greeks have cultivated olive trees and extracted oil from them for centuries. Since then, Olive Oil has been considered a synonym of Greek nutrition.

Agricultural societies that produced Olive oil became comparatively stable. It promoted trade and brought wealth to the olive-growers. However, the need to protect the Greek kingdom and its olive-growing areas had also arisen. In about the 6th century BC, an Athenian legislator called Solon recognized the need to guard this liquid gold. Various Ancient philosophers, physicians, and many historians studied the curative powers of olive oil. They undertook the task of the botanical classification of olives. Even today, scientists are studying the health benefits of olive oil. They are trying to list why the Mediterranean diet is so healthy and nutritious and how it increases the chances of longevity in humans.

Olive Oil and the Social Life

Greece is the place where the first Olympics ever took place. Various facts show the relationship between olive oil and social activities. The winners at the Olympics were honoured with the olive tree branches. Sometimes winners would get massive quantities of olive oil, say five tons. Given the importance of olive oil, we can think of how rich the winner became! When Athens reached its power, the export of olive oil spread across the world. When Rome won over Greece, the Romans learned the secret of olive cultivation and entered the business. The Greek empire has a vast area, explaining why it was a leader in olive production. When the Turks conquered Greece, the cultivation of olives did not stop. It promoted a traditional way of life. The use of olives in religious activities also began. It formed a part of the offerings in the Christian church. Olives were a symbol of peace and love during those times. Olive oil would help light a lamp in the church and form a part of several rites.

After its liberation from the Turks, Greece lost a huge olive cultivation area to the Turks. However, it retained the know-how of qualitative olive production. Since then, Greece has been leading in its production. Greece benefits mainly its geographical location when we talk of olive cultivation. The Mediterranean region has a perfect climate for olive cultivation and has produced the world-famous Greek olive oil. Undoubtedly, Greece is the largest exporter of olive oil. Extra-virgin olive oil, which is the best form of olive oil, is also produced by Greece in large quantities. Every year, Greece makes more than 400,000 tons of olive oil. Greek olive oil is rich in vitamins and is cholesterol-free. Greek olive oil production mainly consists of extra-virgin olive oil, olive oil, and Greek Pomace oil. Greek olive oil is one of the most coveted nutritional products globally.

The olive-cultivators are placed highly in Greece. It is a tradition among the Greeks to plant an olive tree when a child is born. As soon as the child reaches schooling age, the tree is ready to produce its fruit. In essence, the tree grows up with the family and passes from generation to generation. In return for all the love and care that the family showers on the Olive tree, it brings them immense wealth. It produces quality olives that help the family extract the best olive oil. Ancient Greeks believed that the Goddess Athena had created the olive tree with love. That is why the Greeks regard olive trees as high and mighty. Greeks use Olive oil every day for various purposes. The primary use of olive oil is in cooking. It serves the human body with nutrition and health while also keeping the taste of the food.

For centuries, the Mediterranean people have been using olive oil for multiple purposes. Even today, scientists and researchers argue that olive oil is healthy and nutritious for you, chiefly extra-virgin olive oil. Let us look at the potential benefits of olive oil on the human body.

Benefits of Consuming Olive Oil

Olive oil has a lot of benefits for the body, such as:

- **Olive oil is rich in monounsaturated fat**

Olive oil has a generous amount of healthy monounsaturated fat. Fourteen percent of the olive oil is saturated fat. It contains about eleven percent polyunsaturated fat, such as omega-6 and omega-3 fatty acids. Monounsaturated fat called oleic acid forms 73% of the total content in olive oil. Various researches have proved that oleic acid can have a helping effect on inflammation and the genes linked to cancer. Since monounsaturated fat is heat resistant, Olive oil is a healthier choice to consider in cooking.

- **Olive oil is antioxidant-rich**

Olive oil has rich quantities of vitamin E and K and contains many antioxidants. These active antioxidants can reduce the risk of chronic diseases and help keep a person's inflammation and blood cholesterol level in check. Olive oil may even help an individual reduce the risk of various heart diseases.

- **It has many anti-inflammatory properties**

LONG-LASTING INFLAMMATION MAY MAKE a person vulnerable to various diseases such as cancer, diabetes, Alzheimer's, and arthritis. It can even help a person keep their weight in check. Extra-virgin olive oil is rich in anti-inflammatory properties because of the presence of oleic acid. An individual can find all the nutrients that can fight inflammation in olive oil, a one-stop solution for all health problems.

• Olive oil can help reduce the possibility of stroke

The main reason which increases the chances of stroke is the disturbed flow of blood to a person's brain. This disturbance may occur either due to a blood clot or bleeding. Stroke is one of the most common reasons for death among many people. Researchers have been studying the relationship between olive oil and stroke prevention. Time and again, monounsaturated fats have proven to reduce the risk of stroke and heart disease. Olive oil is rich in monounsaturated fats, which form 73% of the total quantity (Estruch et al., 2013).

• It protects a person against heart disease

Heart diseases account for the most common cause of death around the world. Scientists have observed that heart diseases are not quite common in the Mediterranean regions. It has encouraged them to study the Mediterranean diet further. The study proved to reduce the risk of heart diseases (Estruch et al., 2013). Extra-virgin olive oil is the main ingredient of the Mediterranean diet. It helps in lowering the levels of bad cholesterol in the human body. It might even reduce the risk of excessive blood clotting and help in lowering blood pressure.

- **Olive oil helps to keep weight in check**

CONSUMING excessive fats can make a person obese. Extra fats can cause a person to gain weight. Researchers have observed that people in the Mediterranean region have a healthier weight, which led them to study the effects of the Mediterranean diet on a person's weight, finding that olive oil rich in antioxidants has a positive impact (Mendez et al., 2006).

- **Olive oil might help fight Alzheimer's disease**

Alzheimer's is one of the most prevalent neurodegenerative conditions globally and builds various beta-amyloid plaques in an individual's brain cells. A study on mice showed that olive oil could help remove the plagues inside the brain cells (Abuznait et al., 2013). Another study showed that the consumption of olive oil makes a person's brain function better (Martínez-Lapiscina et al., 2013). In addition, studies have shown that olive oil may help reduce the risk of type-2 diabetes (Kastorini & Panagiotakos, 2009) and has positive effects on blood sugar. Olive oil may also help keep the insulin levels in check. Researchers argue that the Mediterranean diet may help keep away the risk of type-2 diabetes by over 40% (Trichopoulou et al., 2000). It is one of the healthiest diets and ranks at the top for its benefits.

- **Its antioxidants have anti-cancer properties**

Many people around the world are at risk of developing cancer. It is a common cause of death among the elderly and adults alike. People in the Mediterranean regions are less likely to have cancer, and many researchers argue that it might be due to extra-virgin olive oil (Trichopoulou et al., 2000). Numerous studies have shown that the compounds in olive oil can help reduce the risk of cancer; they can even fight cancer cells (Menendez et al., 2005). A comprehensive study in this area can help solve this complexity further.

- **Olive oil might help you fight rheumatoid arthritis**

Rheumatoid arthritis is an autoimmune disease that leaves a person with painful and deformed joints. Rheumatoid Arthritis leads your immune system to attack your normal cells by mistake. The anti-inflammatory properties of olive oil help reduce oxidative stress in individuals with rheumatoid arthritis (Kremer et al., 1990). When combined with fish oil, olive oil is an excellent source of anti-inflammatory omega-3 fatty acids.

- **It has many antibacterial properties**

OLIVE OIL IS nutritious because it contains many antibacterial properties that kill bacteria inside a person's body. For example, Helicobacter pylori is a bacteria that lives inside a person's body to cause stomach ulcers and stomach cancer. Various tests have shown that olive oil helps fight the strains of these bacteria, which are otherwise resistant to antibiotics (Romero et al., 2007). A study has proved that if a person consumes at least 30 grams of olive oil every day in their meals, it can help them prevent the harmful effects of Helicobacter pylori in little time (Castro et al., 2012).

What Factors Must You Keep In Mind Before Buying Greek Olive Oil?

Greece is one of the top olive oil-producing countries in the world. Greek olive oil ranks the top among the best oils for health. However, a person must consider a few things before purchasing olive oil because all olive oil is not the same. Here, we will talk about those things. We will also talk about the best kinds of olive oil.

Top Graded Olive Oil

Extra-virgin olive oil is among the top-rated Greek olive oils. First, they take out the oil by pressing the olive. During the process, Greeks make sure not to add any chemicals or hot water. As a result, it has a great aroma, taste, and quality. Greeks derive some 70% of extra-virgin olive oil from their total annual production.

Virgin olive oil also uses the same process for its extraction. However, the quality is comparatively lower to extra-virgin olive oil. Extra virgin olive oil's acidity levels can go up to 2%. It offers a mild aroma and taste, but it is not as exceptional as the extra-virgin olive oil.

While purchasing olive oil, a person must also beware of adulteration. In adulteration, olive oil has a high percentage of refined soyabean oil. Therefore, it can adversely affect your health. An individual can know about adulteration through various tests such as liquid chromatography.

There are various low-grade olive oils available in the market. Pure olive oil is not the right name for the product because it is a blend of soyabean oil and virgin oil. A person might find the products labelled as" 100% pure," but that is not true. It might contain olive oil, but it is not entirely pure but a blend of oils. This kind of oil can hold out against high temperatures, which is why it is the best form of olive oil to use in cooking.

A person must keep in mind to stay away from olive pomace oil. Pomace is the leftover of the olives after they have disposed of good quality olive oil. It is a combination of residue olive oil and virgin olive oil. The quality of Pomace olive oil is poor. It is available at a low price, but individuals must not compromise their health by consuming it.

Colour of Olive Oil

Keeping a view of the colour of olive oil is also of paramount importance. The green colour of the olive oil stipulates that its extraction is from green olives. It usually indicates that these olives were not ripe enough. On the other hand, the extraction of golden-yellow olive oil is from the olives ripening for a long time. Both the green and yellowish olive oils can be extra-virgin olive oil. The cloudy nature of some olive oils is because it has not settled. However, this does not mean that it has cheap quality.

Taste and Smell of Olive Oil

The taste and smell of the oil can help you understand the circumstances of its preparation. A bitter taste indicates that the olives were not ripe enough. A fruity and mild fragrance will tell you that the oil is from ripe olives. You can have a bottle of olive oil entirely based on your preference. If you like a bitter taste, you know which bottle you should choose!

The problem arises when you can not open a bottle of olive oil in the middle of the market to know about its preparation. But, you can tell about its nature after you open it for use at home. If olive oil smells bad, a person should reconsider using it. A poor smell indicates rancidity in the oil and is generally caused due to oxidation and can affect a person in multiple ways.

Acidity Levels

While choosing the right olive oil, a person must also consider acidity levels. Olive oils that have acidity levels below 1% show the best results. The international olive council has a permissible limit of about 3%, but this does not mean that a person should use olive oil with such high concentrations of acids. Extra-virgin olive oil has acidity levels below 1%, which is why it has a good taste and quality. Acidity percentage can determine the quality of olive oil. Therefore, a person must prefer one with low concentrations.

READ the Label

Inspecting before buying is what makes a consumer aware. For example, before purchasing a bottle of olive oil, read the label to find if it's virgin olive oil or extra-virgin olive oil. Also, look for the level of acidity in the oil. The label will also mention the area of origin of the oil; therefore, you can put olive oil from Greece into your shopping bag.

HOW ABOUT TESTING From the Wide Range of Olive Oils?

How does one know if something suits them? It is by testing. Finding the best olive oil for yourself can be a challenging task, so a person can purchase small containers of olive oil from the market to make it an easy task. In this way, an individual can find the best oil for himself by spending a little money. On the other hand, spending money on large bottles of olive oils can be a costly affair. Hence, a person should pick testers to know which oil they like the best. Then, you will thank yourself for buying two bottles of olive oil.

Once a person develops a taste for olive oil, there is no going back! Olive oil serves multiple purposes, and you might want to use it as dressing over your salad or as a sauce. You can even drizzle it over fresh fruits and vegetables. Given all these uses of olive oil, it is always advisable to pick two bottles to avoid any last-minute rush or hindrance to your Mediterranean diet.

Why Do the Greeks Consider Extra-Virgin Olive Oil the Best?

For the past few years, extra-virgin olive oil has become an essential ingredient used in cooking. The discussion about its health benefits is never-ending. Extra-virgin olive oil is highly nutritious and healthy. Greeks use extra-virgin olive oil in large quantities every day. The pungent smell and the bitter taste indicate the oil's health. It keeps a person fit and offers various health benefits to them. However, an individual must keep their eyes open to find any low-quality knock-offs of the olive oil.

Various reports have proved that olive oil has undergone many stages of alteration in today's world. The adulteration levels have been continually increasing. Extra-virgin olive oil is no longer what it claims to be; many people might consider its import from Italy or Greece a stamp on its quality. Recent reports reveal that some countries export more oil than it produces, which raises a question on the credibility of olive oil exporters. It shows that the oil exporters from the top exporting countries mix olive oil with refined soyabean oil.

Lower quality olive oil mixes with chemicals to make the imperfections go away. Some oil producers mix olive oil with cheap vegetable oils and add colourants, and as a result, it looks like olive oil. As a result of this contamination, the market gets flooded with fake extra-virgin olive oil. They offer this diluted extra virgin olive oil at low prices in the market, and, consequently, their demand goes up. They have confused the consumers about the true nature of olive oil. Because of this reason, most consumers do not know what the exact taste of olive oil is.

The Telegraph, in the U.K., reported that four out of five bottles of olive oil from Italy are not pure. With all this confusion and fraud in the olive oil market, it becomes difficult for an individual to pick the right olive oil.

It is always advisable to pick olive oil bottles from the small producers. A person should look for sellers who permit them to taste and smell the oil before purchasing. Authentic extra-virgin olive oil varies in taste and smell depending upon the type of olives picked. It has a fresh fruity fragrance. It can also be grassy or herbal. Sometimes, the extra-virgin olive oil can taste bitter, which does not mean that it is low quality. The bitter taste of olive oil is due to the antioxidants that promote health and help an individual in various ways. The greenish-yellow colour of the olive oil is because of more ripe olives.

It is more buttery, milder, and has a peppery taste. It depends entirely upon the person's preference for which olive oil he picks.

Which Is the Right Place to Buy Olive Oil?

You don't need to visit a farmer's place to buy high-grade olive oil. It won't cost you a fortune either. You can buy extra-virgin olive oil from any small producer or a nearby shop. A person should read the label carefully from whichever shop they plan to buy the olive oil. Greek olive oil is generally the best, and cold pressed extra-virgin olive oil imported from Greece is one of the top-rated oils. Look for the smell and taste of olive oil before purchasing it. Once you select an olive oil that is best for you, you should store it in a proper container to prevent its oxidation. You should keep extra-virgin olive oil in a cool and dry place, and it is advisable to keep it away from the sunlight in a light-proof container. Interaction with light can degrade the quality of the oil. If the oil becomes rancid, it tastes bitter and has a plastic smell. Consuming rancid olive oil is not beneficial for a person's health. Rancid extra-virgin olive oil makes you prone to heart risks and cancer.

Greek olive oil comes in many variants like virgin olive oil, extra-virgin olive oil, and pomace olive oil. It is the pride of the Greeks. Highly valued for its nutritional value, it forms an indispensable part of the Greek and the Mediterranean diet. Olive oil promotes a healthy lifestyle by keeping heart diseases at bay. Its anti-inflammatory properties make it the most recommended oil to use in cooking. Its antioxidant properties are a boon for people. While selecting olive oil, an individual must be cautious about its packaging. People can use dark-coloured containers to protect olive oil from sunlight and rancidity. Olive oil is highly beneficial to help people keep their weight in check. It also proves to be effective in lowering the risk of Alzheimer's and type-2 diabetes. Olive oil is immensely beneficial, and there is no reason why a person should not include this in their regular diet.

7
A BRIEF HISTORY OF THE GREEKS AND THEIR LOVE OF COFFEE

*C*offee is the life of people in Greece. It plays a crucial role in both public and private gatherings. As a result, Greece has embraced coffee in all its forms. From traditional coffee to the exemplary 'frappe,' the history of coffee in Greek culture spans over seven centuries and forms a part of modern society. Our story about the Greek's obsession with coffee begins with the Ottoman empire. The first coffee shop, referred to as 'kafeneio,' opened in 1475 in Constantinople (now Istanbul). With the expansion of the Ottoman empire in Greece, the coffee culture also grew.

As we look at the history of coffee in Greece, by the 17th century, there were more than 300 coffee shops in Thessaloniki alone. With the onset of the 18th century, kafeneio was a well-established Greek institution that served as a destination for good coffee and more social interaction. Greeks go out almost every day for a cup of coffee. Greeks have established a more relaxed and laid-back coffee culture, unlike the people who sip their coffee in a hurry. Traditionally, Greeks hand roasted the green coffee beans in an open pan over the fire. After roasting these coffee beans, they would hand-ground coffee beans in the shop themselves. By the late 19th and 20th centuries, small 'kafekopteio' emerged.

The word kafekopteio means coffee cutter and consists of specialized coffee grinding and roasting shops. The kafekopteio sold historic Greek coffee as well as Tou Briki coffee. The emergence of filter coffee and instant coffee changed the way people consumed the drink. Before this, Greeks followed a long and complex process to make their coffee.

Let us understand the process of evolution of the Greek coffee:

THE 1960s

In the 1960s, the iced version of coffee came into being. It was called frappe and was widely accepted and loved by the Greeks. This change did not mean that the traditional coffee shops shut down, but more modern coffee establishments started to pop up. These contemporary coffee establishments, called cafeterias, gained more momentum among the young Greeks who wanted to socialize. It allowed them to catch up with the present-day American and European culture.

THE 1990s

The beginning of the 1990s marked another coffee wave in Greece. Da Capo café, Italian espresso, and cappuccino entered Greece. Its focal point of the second wave in the 1990s was to provide a refined and rich experience to the Greeks. This time called for the sought-after frappe to refurbish itself into the Freddo. Freddo is, to date, among one of the most consumed coffee by the Greeks. It is an iced version of espresso or cappuccino.

THE 2000s

The already brewing coffee culture among the Greeks reached its peak in the 2000s. Surprisingly, even the global recession did not affect the demand for coffee in Greece. Unemployment could be one reason for the drastic rise in coffee consumption as people spent their leisure time sitting at the coffee shops and indulging in conversations. The general manager of "Kafea Terra" in Greece said that the coffee sales went up instead of declining.

Greek coffee culture has shifted to a new dimension today. There are many varieties of Greek coffee available today; let us look at some of these coffees and their preparation.

Tou Briki or the Greek Coffee

Tou Briki coffee has been a part of Greece's daily consumption for centuries. It is also called Greek coffee and served from a briki, also known as Ibrik, generally a tiny brass pot with a long handle. The secret to preparing Ibrik lies with a single camping gas burner, called gazaki. It is also made on electric stoves or in a machine. But, to truly taste like Greek coffee, it is advisable to prepare it on a single camping gas burner. Ibrik has a rich amount of froth layer on it. This froth layer is known as 'kaimaki' in Greece.

In the ancient days, when the company of women was generally frowned upon by men in various cafeterias, women would prepare the Ibrik at their house and enjoy the beverage. Even today, the Greeks savour Ibrik in full spirits. Ibrik forms a good pair with a sweet dish similar to Turkish delight made with sugar and starch. To prepare Greek coffee, one must follow a rule; it says, "Siga, siga." Siga, Siga translates into slowly, slowly and is self-explanatory. Greeks are known for their patience, and it reflects in their coffee. It takes time and patience to achieve a creamy layer in Ibrik, and it is also advisable to drink the coffee slowly to savour it and prevent you from burning your tongue. Ibrik coffee has ottoman roots. It has a strong, bitter taste, and it leaves a black residue in the bottom of the cup that is not for consumption.

The Frappe

In 1957, the frappe was the most consumed iced coffee in Greece. It is a drink made with soluble coffee, water, and sugar, where it is optional to use sugar and milk. It is a simple beverage to prepare. Anyone can make a frappe at any place. It just requires the mixing of water with instant coffee. One must shake this mixture with strength and add some sugar and milk. The frappe is generally known as the original Greek iced coffee. Interestingly, Dimitris Vakondios, a Greek Nescafe representative, discovered it by a mere accident. Let us have a quick read of Dimitris Vakondios's story:

There was a trade show held at Thessaloniki in Northern Greece in 1957. During his break, Dimitris Vakondios had a sudden urge to drink coffee. There was no hot water available, so he took some granules of coffee and mixed them with cold water. He shook it vigorously and gave birth to what we know as the frappe. During the 1970s, there was a frappe wave in Greece and took on to become the national beverage of Greece. However, it does not form a big part of the Greek coffee culture in the contemporary world. Today, its existence is limited to independent coffee shops and some taverns. Smaller coffee shops and bakeries in Greece prefer to prepare the coffee with espresso machines. A frappe is cheap and an easily accessible coffee. Anyone can make a frappe at home with ease. It is a popular summer drink in Greece and consumed at home when people do not want to step out.

The Freddo

Freddo is the ice version of many espresso beverages. Freddo can be iced espresso, iced cappuccinos, or flat white Freddo. When espresso comes with ice, it becomes a Freddo espresso. Likewise, when a cappuccino comes with ice, it is called a Freddo cappuccino. Freddo is extremely popular in Greece, especially in the summer when temperatures rise, and people crave a cold and a satisfying drink. It is the most commonly consumed iced beverage in Greece. It tastes great, and a customer can get his coffee prepared as per their preference. A consumer can choose among the wide range of options for their Freddo, such as adding cream, milk, soy milk, chocolate, cinnamon, or even letting it be black.

The Freddo came up as an alternative to espresso or Greek coffee when the sales for espresso started tanking. Soaring temperatures were a reason why people started consuming the Freddo. They wanted to have something cool; that is when people started drinking Freddo. Freddo is a double espresso mixed with ice. It became popular in a flash and remains the favourite among the Greeks even today. When you visit Greece, you can see coffee shops almost everywhere. Greeks have an undying love for coffee, and the estimates say that an average Greek consumes nearly 5 kg of coffee every year. This estimate makes Greece the top consumer of coffee in the world.

People in other countries might consider coffee breaks to help them be more productive or catch up with a friend, but in Greece, the coffee breaks play a crucial role in their lives. They consider it as a part of socializing and spending time with themselves. The Greeks like to consume their coffee with a touch of tradition, and they take it very seriously. They drink their coffee with utmost patience. In Greece, having a cup of coffee is known as a very 'Greek' thing to do.

Why do Greek people drink a lot of coffee? Is it healthy? Let us find an answer to these questions about Greek coffee:

GREEK COFFEE and Longevity

Greek coffee promotes a long and healthy life, exciting news for many coffee lovers. Various studies published at *greekcitytimes.com* show that the consumption of Greek coffee could be a link to a long and healthy life. Inquisitive researchers surveyed many elderly Greek residents. They found that those who would consume a cup of boiled Greek coffee or Ibrik showed better cardiovascular health than those who did not. The consumption of an extra cup of Greek coffee reduced the risk of a heart attack by 7 to 8%. It is also said to reduce the risk of stroke. Some findings published in *Vascular Medicine* observed the residents of Ikaria have one of the most extended lifespans in the world. It pointed towards the simple Greek formula that focuses on a cup of coffee per day for this miracle.

A notable difference between Greek coffee and the other caffeine is that Greeks sip coffee slowly. Their attitude towards the coffee is that of patience. Greeks drink their cup of coffee with their friends, family, and at social gatherings. It is distinctly related to various health benefits associated with Greek coffee. The slow pace of drinking coffee is said to reduce the stress levels in the Greeks.

Improved Endothelial Function

Greek coffee shows a better endothelial function than other types of coffee. Endothelial is a thin membrane that lines and protects the blood vessels and the inside of the heart. It functions to release substances that help control vascular relaxation and contraction, as well as enzymes that control blood clotting, immune function, and platelet adhesion.

The endothelial layer breaks down with age and lifestyle habits. For example, various studies show that moderate consumption of coffee every day among the Greeks promotes good endothelial health and brings down the risk of coronary heart disease.

Gerasimos Siasos, a professor at the University of Athens, said, "Boiled Greek type of coffee, which is rich in polyphenols and antioxidants, and contains only a moderate amount of caffeine, seems to gather benefits compared to other coffee beverages."

Helps in Preventing Premature Deaths

Many studies prove that the consumption of Greek coffee may also help prevent premature deaths. The curiosity about the Greek coffee proving to be a miracle drink for a long life led many experts to survey the people on the island of Ikaria. These people drank boiled Greek coffee at least once per day. They had better cardiovascular health when compared to others. These people had been living for over 90 years. Greek coffee is boiled and not filtered. When we bring Greek coffee to boiling, it extracts more nutrients during the process. It has only moderate caffeine because it comprises Arabica coffee, crushed into a fine powder. So, Greek coffee emits more concentrated antioxidants than one's usual cup of coffee. A cup of Greek coffee with a person's meal does wonders to their health.

Greek coffee is also rich in chlorogenic acid, polyphenols, lipid-soluble substances, and other heart-healthy admixtures so that a person's immune system stays healthy. These compounds also help in promoting the health of arteries. As a result, a person has better heart health. Arteries are the transport for the blood to move across a person's body. Therefore, if one starts sipping Greek coffee early from a young age, it could protect them from artery malfunction in their middle and old age.

The boiling method for Greek coffee developed long before people came across filtered coffee. When the fine-grind particles of the Greek coffee boil, it serves as a tasty health punch. It is healthier than a usual cup of American coffee because of the lesser amount of caffeine in every sip. Greeks drink Ibrik about three to five times a day in small cups. Each cup of Ibrik has less than 100 mg of caffeine. Besides the regular Greek coffee, Greeks also feed on a Mediterranean diet. The Mediterranean diet contains some of the most healthy foods and is a reason for their longevity and a healthy heart. Greeks include fresh fruits and vegetables, lean proteins, nuts, seeds, and yogurts in their everyday diet besides Greek coffee.

Coffee stays the most loved beverage across the globe. Even if it is a small grocery run, we never forget to get ourselves a cup of coffee. The secret of Greek coffee to a long life makes a cup of coffee worthwhile. A usual cup of coffee contains kahweol and cafestol and raises cholesterol levels. However, if you have a cup of Greek coffee, it keeps your cholesterol levels in check.

Advantages of Greek Coffee in Your Diet:

When one consumes Greek coffee, it leaves them instantly charged for the day that lies ahead of them. Greek coffee comes with a plethora of health benefits. The slow sipping of Greek coffee helps relieve stress and leaves a person feeling refreshed and energized. Greek coffee's health benefits are not limited to offering long life. It has many additional health benefits that should find space in our discussion. Let us look at the benefits of making Greek coffee a part of our everyday routine:

- **It helps in promoting weight loss**

As popularised by Dr. Bob Arnot in his book, the coffee diet claims that drinking Greek coffee several times a day can help boost a person's metabolism. He pointed out that the people living on the Greek island of Ikaria consume around 720 ml of coffee every day. It adds up to three cups of coffee per day. He further states that the long life of the Greeks is because of the high intake of antioxidant-rich Greek coffee. Bob Arnot's coffee diet recommends a person consume 1,500 calories every day. This diet includes at least three cups of coffee that one must drink. Therefore, Greek coffee can help people increase their metabolism and make weight loss easy.

- **Greek coffee leaves you with healthy arteries**

Inflammation in the arteries can leave a person at risk of various health problems. This is because the arteries act as a transporting agent for the blood. Therefore, reducing the risk of cardiovascular diseases as early as possible can help one maintain good health in middle age. On the other hand, calcification of the arteries can cause the heart to function poorly. As already discussed before, Greek coffee is rich in chlorogenic acid, polyphenols, and lipid-soluble substances. Its heart-healthy substances help in protecting the arteries.

- **It helps protect a person from heart attacks and strokes**

Now we know how Greek coffee promotes the health of the arteries. When the arteries function correctly, the blood circulation improves in an individual's body.

Many people are at risk of heart attacks and strokes because of poor blood flow. Consumption of Greek coffee helps a person ensure better blood circulation and helps to keep the risk of heart attacks and strokes at bay.

- **It improves overall cardiovascular health and boosts immunity**

Dr. Mehmat, a cardiologist, states that Greek coffee might help you increase your cardiovascular health (Dr. Mehmat, n.d.). Greek coffee is rich in antioxidants and enhances cardiovascular health, leaving one with a healthy heart.

- **Boosts the mood of a person**

All types of coffee are known to boost the mood of a person. Greek coffee is not an exception to this statement. Moderate consumption of Greek coffee every day can help a person relieve stress and acts as a mood booster. Furthermore, since people drink Greek coffee, it helps them develop patience. Also, going out for a cup of Greek coffee in a cafe or boiling it in your kitchen with your friends and family enables you to connect more. It makes you a sociable person and boosts a person's mood immediately.

Reduces the risk of diabetes

The presence of chlorogenic acids in Greek coffee serves as a deterrent to diabetes. Greek coffee helps in stabilizing a person's blood sugar levels. It is known to reduce inflammation and fat accumulation in a person's body, hence reducing the risk of diabetes. A Mediterranean diet works wonders for a person prone to diabetes (Martín-Peláez et al., 2020b). Greek coffee forms a part of the rich Mediterranean diet and helps prevent type 2 diabetes.

Is Greek Coffee Different From Your Usual Cup of Coffee?

The next question in your mind is whether Greek coffee is different from the regular filter coffee that we consume in our day-to-day lives. Well, Greek coffee is indeed a little different from our regular coffee. Let us look at the reasons that put Greek coffee at the top:

1. To prepare a cup of Greek coffee, we boil the ground powder. Boiling the coffee powder will help absorb more nutrients from the coffee to offer many health benefits. On the other hand, we do not always do the same when a regular coffee brews.

2. Greek coffee powder is made with Arabica coffee beans. The Greek coffee beans are rich in antioxidants. Other coffee brands might not offer a coffee so rich in antioxidants, which help flush the harmful oxidizing agents from one's body. However, the agents have the potential to damage the human body.

3. Greek coffee has some of the most significant compounds lacking in other coffee brands. It

explains the wide prevalence of Greek coffee culture.

Where Can One Enjoy Greek Coffee?

Greece is a heaven for lovers of coffee. Coffee is so intertwined with the people of Greece that a coffee shop is not hard to find. Many bars in Greece serve coffee during the day. These shops have availability for all sorts of Greek coffee, ranging from Ibrik to Freddo. However, if one wants to enjoy classic Greek coffee, it is advisable to visit a local independent coffee shop in Greece. The secret to savouring Greek coffee lies in drinking it slowly and enjoying every sip of it. Many bakeries also have a coffee machine to sell coffee to their customers.

Greek coffee, known for its health wonders, is popular among all age groups. It is no less than a miracle that Greek coffee promotes long life. It is easily accessible and does not require rocket science to prepare it. A wide range of greek coffee is available in the market, including pure arabica coffee. The preparation of Greek coffee involves boiling the coffee. It ensures that the maximum nutrients absorb from it. Its antioxidant-rich properties make Greek coffee a part of the Mediterranean diet. Sipped slowly and patiently, Greek coffee serves as a foundation to build social relationships among the people in Greece. The Greeks consider their coffee culture a tradition and not a mere moment to drink coffee. It acts as a stress buster and promotes the health of the heart. The heart-healthy Greek coffee has no reason why one should not welcome it in their life.

8
GREEK HOLISTIC HEALTH WITH HERBS

Nature has always been the provider for us, whether it's about food or medicine. Some diseases can easily be cured with the help of medical plants and herbs. The ancient Greeks were also considered the ancestors of modern medicine. Despite being underestimated as simply seasonings, herbs are an essential element of making the Mediterranean Diet so tasty and nutritious. In ancient Greek medicine, they also perform a unique role. Hippocrates, the "Father of Medicine," used almost 250 different herbs local to his native land of Kos in his practice. Medical technology has become less reliant on Mother Nature to help heal and well-being. Yet, there is a renewed interest in the miraculous health effects of these remarkable plants. The wide use of herbs is also inextricably linked to Greek cuisine. In this chapter, we'll look at the history of

THE HOLISTIC GREEK DIET & WAY OF LIFE

our favourite herbs and how they became prominent in the rest of the world. These herbs are endemic to Greece and are mainly grown wild on rocky outcroppings, filling the air with their lovely scents. Though modern medicine has progressed, several diseases could be easily cured with traditional medical science (*Examine the Theatre*, n.d.). The ancient Greeks can assist us in thinking about contemporary concerns that are important to treat infections with the help of modern or old remedies.

Diet, medication, and operations were the three main focuses of ancient Greek medicine. And diet was always the priority. That doesn't mean the diet is only about what you eat or drink; it's more about your everyday routine and your entire way of life. Including how much you exercised, total hours of sleep, what kind of food you are eating, and if you've exercised more than your potential, in addition to how much time you spend making yourself happy. Health is defined as the balancing of fluids throughout the body. And it wasn't simply the way of living that affected one's equilibrium. It also depended on how someone's body interacted with the outside world.

With problems like weight and mental health occupying so much of a doctor's attention these days, the environment may be pretty important. In such a situation, it's crucial to consider how the Ancient Greeks approached human health holistically since it's pretty evident that medicine needs faith. In the ancient era, doctors generally treated individuals with suspicion. As they think when someone is sick, they get access to one's body and can do whatever they want, and that issue is quite reasonable; since there were no such equipment or rules and regulations that could help patients if they suffer from something else. The patient and doctors were also strangers to one another. Furthermore, simply being unwell for a male demonstrated a lack of manhood. Therefore, it's hard to allow somebody to treat or check your body whom you might trust with your health during that time was considered quite dangerous.

A doctor's appearance must be clean to acquire a patient's faith. It's all about the white coat today. There was also the matter of dressing simply, avoiding heavy odours, and never reciting poetry at the patient's bedside. You'll understand why if you've already read a Greek tragedy. (*Examine the Theatre*, n.d.-b). When you're sick, hearing someone utter things like "Alone in my pain, I would crawl, clutching my horrible foot" isn't exactly pleasant.

The use of herbal medicines for treatment is as old as humans. The link between humans and their hunt for natural therapies runs back thousands of years, as demonstrated by many sources, including ancient writings, historical structures, and sometimes even natural plant remedies. The understanding of medicinal plant implementation results from several years of fighting against diseases. As a result, man learned to seek medications in plant barks, seeds, fruit bodies, and other components (Petrovska, 2012). Modern scientific knowledge has recognized their dynamic function, and this has included a variety of plant-based medications known to ancient cultures and utilized for centuries into modern pharmacotherapy. The potential of healthcare practitioners to tackle the challenges that have arisen with the distribution of professional services in the facilitation of man's life has enhanced as knowledge of the innovation of concepts related to the use of medicinal herbs, and the advancement of recognition has improved.

Herbs have always played a significant part in medicine, dating back to the first recorded occurrences. By Dioscorides (Daisy, 2017), a Greek physician and a botanist who published widely on the area, to Hippocrates, the "Father of Modern Medicine," early healthcare professionals recognized and supported the relevance of herbal treatments. Medicine was not yet a defined discipline in ancient Greece's initial periods. Over time, experts from several professions applied their expertise to health, leading to medicine as a discipline.

The ancient Greeks were always eager for philosophy and logic-based debates, and thus a desire to understand why things were possible or things occurred. This natural curiosity opened up the door for dramatic improvements in science and mathematics.

According to ancient documents, in 700 BC, they established an ancient medical school in Cnidus. They started studying ill people in this school (Murrell, 2018). Alcmaeon, a teacher at this institution, lived approximately 500 BC and published several books on medicine, despite being most likely a philosopher of science instead of a physician. He believed to be the pioneer to embrace the idea of internal factors of sickness. He claimed that illness might be caused by environmental issues, poor diet, and a sedentary lifestyle. As Greek doctors began to ponder if all diseases and disorders had a natural source, they began to contemplate treating disease with natural treatments. Until then, the most common type of medicine had only been incantations or efforts to fight against demonic possession.

Alexander the Great transformed Greece into a vast empire that spanned the Middle East around 300 BC. The Greeks created Alexandria in Egypt, transforming it into a significant educational and intellectual hub. The Ancient Greeks still trusted in and also adored their gods. However, science became extremely important as they attempted to describe the causes and cures to illnesses and other lifestyle sectors.

Ancient Greece embraced not just the land we

know today but also Greeks residing throughout the Mediterranean, especially Italy, Sicily, and the westernmost parts of modern-day Turkey (HHRN, 2017). Furthermore, the Hellenistic and Roman dynasties had individuals from a wide range of geographical locations and cultures, all of which impacted medicine at the time. It is commonly acknowledged that ancient Greeks created the pillars of science and the study of physiology, anatomy, and psychology to discover the causes of illnesses and improve health status. There were also the moral responsibilities of persons working in health and science. As medical research progressed, distinct perspectives on medical practice emerged due to several medical schools. Knidos doctors' viewpoint is one of the most well-known, concentrating only on the ailment that afflicted the patient (Kleisiaris et al., 2014b). However, the Methodists' (medical thought) philosophy, created by Asclepius and centred on sustaining health and the necessity of knowing the entire evaluation of sufferers' health and medical condition, has become the most popular philosophy thus far.

The Holistic Healing Philosophy

Ancient Greek and Roman medicine and healing techniques generally relied on the use of herbs, meals, and nutrition as medicinal aids; however, wines, meat, and dairy, as well as minerals and clays, too were utilized (HHRN, 2017b). But before the Hippocratic Corpus (c. 450-350 BC), allusions to gods or men curing with plants may be discovered in Homeric Hymns as well as Homeric epics from the 8th century BC, as well as oral traditions from far earlier. Physical artifacts at places like castles, funeral chambers, crockery, vases, and wall paintings, among others, provide evidence of medical plants in Greek culture (Anon, n.d.-a). According to Greek medicine's holistic healing philosophy, man is fundamentally a product of nature or the natural world. When a person is connected or lives in harmony with nature, they increase their lifespan, and also, whenever the connection and equilibrium break down from nature, it leads to sickness. Healing is the process of regaining the equilibrium and balance that has been lost. For thousands of years, humans and all the other living beings on earth have grown and flourished inside this all-encompassing ecosystem, depending on it for their medication, existence, and nutrition. Whenever animals in the forest become ill or unwell, they would start chewing or eating on certain medicinal plants until they felt healthier. Humans' herbal remedies arose from a desire to emulate the animal kingdom's global healing technique.

The ancient Greeks realized the importance of physical and social circumstances and individual behaviour in maintaining good health. They described health as inner and outer dynamic balance (Anon, 2017). They also considered the physical and social health determinants, the empowerment of persons and communities with new political or participatory organizations, and a focus on medical literacy and skill enhancement. They also understood the value of supporting settings and sound public policies and reshaped medicine to be more realistic and humanistic. Herbal remedies are a global practice across all of the world's traditional systems of medicine that produce herbal treatment processes or strategies based on their holistic healing ideas and conceptions. Greek medicine is nothing like this rule. Its unique herbal medicine system is based on its four central beliefs:

- The four basic qualities
- The four elements
- The four humors
- The four temperaments

The actual specifics of Greek medicine's herbal healing approach evolved through years of clinical practice among Greek medics. According to the Greek medicine system, all kinds of herbal medicine systems should be effective and have both practical and theoretical components. The theory is required to guide the doctor's views and assumptions in developing a diagnosis and treatment plan. On the other hand, to pick the correct herbs and treatments that truly work, one must have practical knowledge, either one's own or that of one's professors.

Hippocrates advises against allowing theory to get ahead of clinical practice and creates outcomes in his writings. "Foolish the doctor who despises the knowledge acquired by the ancients," he added, highlighting the significance of heritage as well as a sensible approach.

According to medicine and science, everything in the world has its fundamental character and temperament or harmony of the four essential qualities (greekmedicine.net, n.d.):

- Hot
- Cold
- Wet
- Dry

That's how Greek medicine examines the nature and quality of herbs. Next, Galen devised a four-degree metric system for each of the four essential qualities to more precisely measure how hot, cold, wet, or dry a plant was—allowing the doctor and pharmacist to develop and prescribe medications with greater precision.

To put the body back into equilibrium, herbalists typically utilize medicines whose natures are opposite or complementary to the characteristic of the illness. For example, eliminating herbs with properties that are dramatically opposed to offending humor are utilized to decrease or distribute them in vast amounts or overflow cases. Likewise, tonic herbs contain properties or natural extracts that the body lacks or requires to regain health and completeness in deficient circumstances. Since they discovered that the body and brain should be in harmony, the ancient Greeks thought mental and physical wellness were connected (Petrovska, 2012). According to Aristotle, athletics and gymnastics are necessary for the growth of the individual physique to maximize the functional capability and balance among brain and body, as evidenced by the famous statement "healthy brain in a healthy body."

Ancient herbs in Greece are still used for healing the body. Like any other ancient herbal medicinal system, Greek herbal medicine employs the principle of herbal flavours and energetics to develop therapeutic identification and utilization of herbs. Here are some identification and utilization of herbs in the Greek herbal medicine (greekmedicine.net, n.d.):

Stomachics are any herbs that help the stomach and gastrointestinal system in any manner. Bitter stomachics are soothing and cleansing, and they're used to treat warm, inflammatory, hyperacidity, and bilious stomach problems. In sluggishness and congestion, scented stomachics gently balance and accelerate gastrointestinal function. Pungent stomachics are considerably warmer and much more vigorous in action, quickly removing excess coldness and phlegm. Anodynes, out of the different types of pain-relieving herbs, unwind and disperse muscle cramps with their gentle warming and dispersing operation.

Also, roots were one of the medical treatments used by Greeks. For example, Epimenides of Crete (7th/6th century BC), a semi-mythical philosopher, seer, and poet, is claimed to have successfully cleaned an Athens accused of sacrilege during the Cylonian Affair (632 BC) when a failed revolution resulted in a slaughter outside a temple (Davias, 2019). The poet is also famous for his herbal combination known as 'alimon,' which he consumed in moderate doses every day to avoid feeling hungry. Other notable members of the magical-mythical group of root cutters were the centaur Chiron, Achilles' instructor; the curing deity Asclepius; the sorceress Circe; the soothsayer-healer Melampous; and Machaon and Podaleirios, Asclepius' physician-sons who fought in the Trojan War.

Roots were important in ancient Greek medicine not just because of their medicinal properties but also because of their symbolic value. They were created inside the embraces of all nutrition and goodness of the Earth's Goodess and served as excel-

THE HOLISTIC GREEK DIET & WAY OF LIFE

lent tools for body and soul recovery. Furthermore, due to these beneath travels, the sacred snake understood all of the roots' mysteries and could apply them to the countless patients' advantage. Therefore, they came to Asclepius' healing sanctuaries (Asclepias) to be cleaned and cured. Here are some of the most coveted roots utilized by ancient Greek healers. With all stressors of contemporary life and health issues that come with them, some of these cures may once again be effective.

The marshmallow (Althaea Officinalis) is grown in many places because even people that aren't interested in its medicinal properties are wowed by the abundance of blooms it produces every spring. The plant's most prominent attribute, even so, is its remarkable medicinal properties, as reported by Dioscorides in "De Materia Medica," who writes: "It is named althaea due to its many healing powers and its multidimensionality of uses," the name sourced from the ancient Greek verb althaino, which means "to heal." (Daisy, 2017). Ancient Greek medics used to mix the root with grape juice and then administer the resultant wine to cure injuries and blisters after a time of fermentation. They also thought that preparing it as a decoction was helpful in various medical ailments, including dysuria, sciatica, dysentery, and kidney stones.

The making of salep, a classic beverage for alleviating coughs and calming stomach pains, is an

Eastern craft that became well-known in Greek territories during the Ottoman period. It's made from the tubers of a lovely orchid called the early purple orchid (Orchis mascula), which very few people know was prized in ancient Greece. It was given the name orchis after just a young person who has been the son of a nymph and a satyr. The impetuous adolescent misbehaved and snatched the virtue of one of Dionysus' maidens one particular night at an orgiastic ceremony in his honour. The god's female worshippers, the maenads, tore him to bits almost immediately. His father begged Dionysus to spare him and bring him back to life in his grief. The underground section of this plant was thought to have extraordinary characteristics in prehistoric days, most likely due to its likeness to male genitalia. Dioscorides first conveyed an ancient faith about sernikovotano, as the orchid is now commonly known in Greece, and it has been maintained nearly unaffected in many areas: Particularly regarding, though, that the big root, food consumed by men, produces male offspring and the relatively small roots, eaten by women, produce female children.

The root of the herb elecampane (Inula helenium), which Theophrastus refers to as "Chiron's panacea" and included in the medicinal arsenal of the centaur Chiron, was yet another cure used by ancient healers. It reappears four centuries later in Dioscorides' works when he refers to it as 'elenion.'

Helen's tears, according to legend, originated from her grief over the loss of her helmsman on her trip to Egypt with Menelaus after the fall of Troy. Elecampane root was used in a variety of ways in ancient medicine. Physicians used it to cure spasms, sneezing, flatulence, and the detrimental consequences of wild animal attacks by boiling it in honey or making a medicinal wine. It was regarded as a good remedy with advantages for the gastrointestinal and respiratory systems. For ages, the root of larger burdock (Arctium lappa), also known as 'arkeion' and 'Prosopis,' was used to cure various medical issues. It was used to heal burns, snake bites, and internal aches as a decoction in hemoptysis (coughing up blood) with abscesses or as a juice combined with honey to cure burns, snake bites, and internal pains of the ancient Greeks.

However, it was principally used locally to ease the pain and inflammation of injuries and to cure chilblains and infections after being produced by heating in wine or by a basic, vigorous crushing. It was crushed, combined with salt, and applied to severe injuries caused by rabid dog bites. These wounds recovered more rapidly in this manner, but without lessening the risk of the deadly illness being passed to the bite victim in any way. In Greek medicines (greekmedicine.net, n.d.), inventive and effective herbal concoctions are employed in therapy, all of which are designed to provide maximal healing power to the location of the illness. Herbal teas, tablets, and powders are mixed and matched with various common treatments on hand, such as syrups and tinctures. Compresses, liniments, salves, cataplasms or poultices, and fermentations are external or topical treatments.

According to anthropologists (Murrell, 2018), people employed medicinal plants in prehistoric times. According to some evidence, they may have used plants and natural things as remedies. However, it's challenging to say the complete range because plants decompose quickly.

We may assume that many curative herbs or plants would've been native to the area, though it was not always the situation. Nomadic tribes might have access to a wider variety of materials because they travelled long distances. According to data from modern archaeological sites in Iraq, Mallow and yarrow were utilized around 60,000 years ago.

The herb yarrow (Achillea millefolium) is an astringent, diaphoretic, fragrant, and stimulant (Murrell, 2018). Astringents assist in stopping bleeding by causing tissues to constrict and presumably administered to wounds, cuts, and abrasions. A diaphoretic is a moderate fragrance that stimulates perspiration. It may also possess anti-inflammatory, anti-ulcer, and antipathogenic effects. Yarrow is still used today to heal wounds, respiratory infections, digestive issues, skin diseases, and liver illness worldwide.

Documentation of rosemary usage as a therapeutic herb has been found in numerous parts of the world and is credited with various medical properties across the globe. Consequently, it's difficult to say what it was used for in ancient times (Murrell, 2018). The honeybees adore the scented blooms of lemon balm (Melissa officinalis), thus the Latin botanical name (Melissa is Greek for honeybee). Honey was first found by a group of nymphs known as melissa in ancient mythology. The herb is well-known for its ability to soothe the heart and boost the soul during times of stress, and it can help anyone suffering from anxiety, melancholy, sleeplessness, or panic attacks. It also contains antiviral qualities that are effective against herpes and shingles. In De Materia Medica, Dioscorides cites its usage as a wine-infused liniment (Christodoulou, 2019).

Because it grows wild over Greece's mountainsides, Tsai Tou Vounou (Sideritis) is known as mountain tea. It was known as ironwort in ancient times because it was used to treat wounds caused by iron weapons during war. "He who is made of iron," in Greek, means "he who is formed of iron." The whole herb is traditionally used in an infusion (short boiling time), which can help to strengthen the immune system, aid digestion, and prevent colds (Christodoulou, 2019).

In Greek, bay leaf (Laurus nobilis L.) is called Dafni, from the tale of Apollo following the indifferent nymph Daphne. The gods provided her sanctuary from Apollo by changing her into a bay tree to answer her pleas. Heartbroken Apollo later personified the tree in honour of love-shorn poets. Bay leaves were used to form crowns for monarchs, battle heroes, and Olympians in ancient Greece and Rome and were supposed to protect against sickness and evil spirits. High-dose bay leaf tea may have been used by priestesses at the Temple of Delphi to induce a trance state and divine the gods' intent (Christodoulou, 2019).

While specific old herbal medicine treatments are no longer employed for apparent causes, such as deadly battle wounds or dangerous snake bites, the therapeutic virtues of these plants have not altered (Christodoulou, 2019). It's fascinating to envision our ancient Greek forefathers gathering leaves for the same tea we may drink now, all while basking in the same brilliant Mediterranean sun and revelling in the delight of living in a land rich in healing traditions. "Custom is king," as Herodotus (484-425 BCE), the father of history, famously said.

RECIPES

Avgolemono Soup
(Choice of chicken, beef, or no meat)

- 1 package of chicken legs
- 1 small onion, finely chopped
- ¼ cup of orzo, rice, or millet (your choice)
- 4 tbsp olive oil
- Salt and Pepper

What you need to make the Avgolemono Sauce:

- 2 eggs
- ¼ cup lemon juice

If you are using chicken, remove the skin and discard. Be sure to wash the chicken under cold running water. Place in a large pot and add 2 pints water. Bring to a boil; skim the access froth on the pot as it boils. Once the chicken is fully cooked, remove it from the broth. Set aside.

Add the olive oil, onions, and your choice of rice, orzo or millet to the pot. Cover and reduce the heat and simmer for about 20 minutes until orzo, rice, or millet is tender. While simmering, take your chicken and cut it into small cubes. Add to your pot and simmer for another 10-15 minutes. Remove from heat.

How to make the avgolemono sauce and add it to the soup:

Take both eggs and separate the yokes from the egg whites.

Place the egg white in a separate bowl and beat with an electric beater until it becomes frothy. Add the two egg yolks to your mixture and continue to beat with a fork. Add your lemon juice.

Take a latel and slowly add some of the contents of your broth to your avgolemono mixture. Try not to grab pieces of chicken. Add a few times with the latel. Mix everything together. Sprinkle the soup with freshly ground pepper and salt and serve hot.

If you prefer to not use meat, you can make a broth with vegetables of your choosing and then follow the avgolomeno technique.

Greek Lentil Soup

- 1 cup lentils (preferably the small brown lentils)
- 1 onion
- 2 whole garlic cloves
- 2 bay leaves
- 1 small fresh tomato
- 2 tbsp tomato paste (mix with some water until blended)
- 4 tbsp olive oil
- 1 teaspoon oregano
- Salt and pepper to taste
- 3 tbsp vinegar

Wash and pick over the lentils. Add about 2 pints of water, onions, garlic, fresh tomato, tomato paste, and olive oil to a large pot and boil. Add lentils, bay leaves and oregano, cover and simmer for about 45 minutes or until lentils are tender.

Once lentils are to your desired tenderness, lower the heat, add vinegar, sprinkle with ground pepper and salt, serve hot or cold and accompany with a side of olives.

Mbirgiami (Eggplant & Zuchinni Bake)

- 1 large eggplants cut into thick layers
- 1 large zuchinni cut into thick layers
- 2 potatoes
- 1 onion, chopped
- 3 garlic cloves, crushed
- 2 tbsp parsley
- ½ tsp dill
- 1 fresh crushed tomato
- 1 cup olive oil
- 1 tbsp oregano
- salt and pepper
- 1/3 cup feta

Layer eggplant, zuchinni, potatoes, chopped onion, crushed garlic, tomato, parsley and dill into a large cooking pan and mix. Add olive oil and about a cup of water to the mixture, and sprinkle with oregano. Bake at 350 degrees for approximately 30-45 minutes. Sprinkle with feta, salt and pepper and serve hot.

Spanakorizo (Spinach and Rice)

- 1 package of spinach
- ¼ cup rice
- 1 onion diced
- 2 green onions chopped
- ½ cup olive oil
- 1 tbsp parsley
- ½ tsp dill
- Salt and pepper

Wash the spinach and trim off the stems. Chop the spinach and blanch it in boiling water. Drain and set aside. In a large pot, saute onions with some olive oil, and add water, spinach, green onions, parsley, dill, and rice. Simmer and cover for about 15-20 minutes until the rice is tender and has absorbed most of the water. Do not stir the mixture while cooking. Turn off the heat. Add salt and pepper to taste.

Can be served hot or cold and accompanied with feta cheese and olives.

AFTERWORD

Health can be defined in several different ways, and it's usually divided into a series of figures and classifications that don't always reflect what a healthy balanced body and mind seem like. While contemporary western medicine has made many remarkable and life-saving improvements, one of its flaws is its segregated aspect of health, which focuses on the body in segments of specific symptoms and components rather than the whole system. That's why holistic health is so essential: To achieve proper optimum health in the physical, emotional, and spiritual senses, we must perceive and nurture the body as the remarkable system it is.

Ancient health practices in China and India, dating back 5,000 years, emphasized a healthy lifestyle in sync with nature. During the 20th century, holistic principles fell out of favour in Western nations. The concept of health shifted dramatically as a result of scientific medical advancements. Being healthier became a process of using synthesized medications to destroy microscopic invaders. People thought they could live easily with poor lifestyle choices since medical technology would 'fix' them as problems occurred. On the other hand, medical treatments are more detrimental than sickness in some cases.

Furthermore, many chronic illnesses do not respond to conventional treatments. Therefore, people go back to the holistic way and health to find better options. The holistic living approach grows in popularity every year, as holistic concepts provide practical solutions to the growing demand for improved health and well-being.

With changes in climate affecting our surroundings more and more every day, we must have a systematic way of tackling health concerns in the future. Holistic health also considers the several internal and external environment aspects that may support or affect our health and well-being. It works on the five basic principles—Physical, mental/emotional, intellectual, social, and spiritual well-being. This encompasses physical health, psychological well-being, mental stimulation, work-related stress, financial stress, relationship anxiety, social stress levels, and spiritual stressors. Hippocrates, the ancient Greek Father of Medicine, wrote that "all

AFTERWORD

diseases begin in the gut" and that we must "let medicine be thy food and food thy medicine" for real healing and optimal health, and that "natural forces within us are the true healers of disease." A diet in Ancient Greece was all about better health, and food was a big part of that. The mind, body, and spirit needed to be nurtured for good health. The diet was an essential factor in maintaining gut health and a robust immune system. The Ancient Greeks also recognized the link between good health and emotional and mental well-being.

"Wisdom healing" was the ancient Greek Hippocratic approach of health, which involved using food to help the body, mind, and soul. It is crucial to eat a variety of foods beneficial to our health while limiting or avoiding detrimental ones. It starts with cooking and eating fresh, unprocessed, and unfiltered ingredients and foods. For instance, eating fresh certified organic fruits and vegetables (particularly greens and living grains like sprouts), organic supplements including spirulina, herbs, and spices, herbal teas, filtered water, good quality oils such as olive oil, avocado oil, and coconut oil is what the holistic Greek diet is all about. In addition, eat raw seeds and nuts, raw chocolate, fermented foods, natural sweeteners such as fresh honey, maple syrup, lentils, grains including couscous, buckwheat, amaranth, brown rice, spelled, and barley, and combine omega-3 to omega-6 fats into your diet.

AFTERWORD

The ancient Greeks used meditation, prayer, food therapy, massage therapy, sun therapy, and exercise therapy to help emotional wellness. Aristotle, for example, recognized the healing effect of music, and several physicians in ancient Greece used frequency to promote digestion, cure mental problems, and improve sleep.

Bread, olive oil, wine, and greens summed up the ancient Greek diet. While the wealthier Greeks could explore a wide range of cuisines, these four items were the staples of their diet. They ate homemade wheat or barley bread for breakfast, lunchtime, and dinner often dunked in wine. This traditional meal was accompanied by fruit, vegetables, or legumes, two of which were flavoured with spices, herbs, and olive oil. The Greeks often had nuts and a lot of seafood; their preferred beverage was wine, which they drank at all three meals, including breakfast, but mixed with water to make it less potent. Pheasant and quail were among the poultry bred by the ancient Greeks, but the birds were cherished more for their eggs than meat. Red meat was scarce; therefore, the Greeks ate lean meat like pig, rabbit, and goat when they did eat it. The ancients, unlike contemporary Europeans, did not cook with butter or milk, but they did eat cheese, honey, figs, and fermented dairy products comparable to current Greek yogurt.

The Greeks consumed a lot of olive oil. This

custom lasted until only a few decades ago when the Greeks started eating a more Americanized cuisine of imported fast food and prepackaged items. Prior to that, Greeks consumed more olive oil than everyone else in the world, including elsewhere in the Mediterranean. Olive oil, which is high in healthy fat, is the key to reducing body fat, making you feel full, raising your body's metabolism and capacity to oxidize fat, all while lowering your risk of heart disease and improving your general health.

Jump a few thousand years forward: Based on what the residents of Crete ate in the 1950s and 1960s, the ancient Greek diet is known today as the Mediterranean diet. We term this diet the Greek diet to distinguish it from ineffectual and hybridized variants of the conventional Mediterranean diet.

We understand that the "Mediterranean diet" was the core of their diet. Olives, grapes, and wheat were the most readily accessible crops. The ancient Greeks were active people who regarded food for function as much as joy, as indicated by their nutrition and athletic achievements. According to holistic health concepts, health entails more than not getting sick. One popular idea is to think of well-being as a continuous line. The line depicts all possible health levels. Premature death is represented by the left end of the line. The highest potential degree of well-being, or optimum well-being, is at the far right end. The line's center point represents the absence of visible sickness. All levels of disease are now assigned to the left half of the health spectrum. The right side demonstrates that there is still a lot of space for growth even when no disease appears to be present. Holistic health is a process that never ends. As a way of life, it entails making an emotional commitment to be on the right side of the health spectrum. People can improve their health regardless of their existing health situation.

The use of herbal medicines for treatment is as old as humans. The link between humans and their hunt for natural medicines runs back thousands of years, as demonstrated by many sources, including ancient writings, historical structures, and sometimes even natural plant remedies. Understanding medicinal plant implementation results from several years of fighting against diseases. As a result, man learned to seek medications in plant barks, seeds, fruit bodies, and other components. Modern scientific knowledge has recognized their dynamic function, and this has included a variety of plant-based medications known to ancient cultures and utilized for centuries into modern pharmacotherapy. The potential of healthcare practitioners to tackle the challenges that have arisen with the distribution of professional services in the facilitation of man's life has enhanced as knowledge of the innovation of concepts related to the use of medicinal herbs, and the advancement of recognition has improved.

AFTERWORD

Eating with peace, calmness, and happiness is another key eating behaviour for a healthy gut and better immunity. It's crucial not to rush through meals. When we speed up our mealtime, we disrupt the balance, the energy flow, and the time required to savour a meal that will nurture and rejuvenate our body and spirit in the end. We must all eat thoughtfully and become mindful of our foods to live a healthy life. We also have to pay attention to how our food influences our mood.

In conclusion, it is essential to eat and think to nurture our mind, body, and soul. Include probiotic foods and eat meals free of toxins and chemicals, precisely as they did in the Greek Culture. To maintain healthy, cheerful mind and emotions, do things that bring you joy; and, of course, get some workouts done daily. According to Hippocrates, if we could give each person the right amount of diet and physical activity, not too little and not too much, we would've discovered the best path to health.

The Greek Diet does all of this while focusing on the "pleasure factor," or how much we love foods. No weight-loss program should make you forego the flavours, sensations, and impacts of nourishing meals and beverages that we believe make life worthwhile. Have a cup of coffee for breakfast and a glass of wine for dinner, as well as dessert. To live a healthy life, you don't need to eliminate carbs, gluten, or other foods, nor do you need to watch calories or limit your consumption. The key to effective and long-term weight management is feeling happy, energetic, and confident about yourself and whatever you eat—not starving, unhappy, and deprived.

References

8 Rules We Can Learn From the Greek Diet and Lifestyle. (2015, August 23). Lifehack. https://www.lifehack.org/293697/8-rules-can-learn-from-the-greek-diet-and-lifestyle

Brazier, Y. (2018, November 9). *Ancient Greek medicine: Influences and practice.* Www.medicalnewstoday.com. https://www.medicalnewstoday.com/articles/323596#culture-and-philosopy

Bread in Ancient Greece. (n.d.). Ελληνικό Πρωϊνό. Retrieved December 17, 2021, from https://www.greekbreakfast.gr/story/bread-in-ancient-greece/?lang=en

Bread: more than just food! (2018, June 18). Griekse Les | Lato Cultuur Centrum. https://griekse-les.nl/bread-more-than-food/

Christodoulou, M. (2019). *Medicinal Herbs in Ancient Greece.* The Greek Herbalist. https://www.thegreekherbalist.com/herbalcolumn/medicinalherbsinancientgreece

daisy. (2017, November 17). *The Uses of Plants in Medicine in Ancient Greece and Rome.* Www.r-cpe.ac.uk. https://www.rcpe.ac.uk/heritage/talks/uses-plants-medicine-ancient-greece-and-rome

Davias, O. (2019, February 21). *They Were Right: 7 Medicinal Plants Used by Ancient Greek Physicians.* Greece Is. https://www.greece-is.com/they-were-right-7-medicinal-plants-used-by-ancient-greek-physicians/

Doyle, I. (2021). *How to Eat Like an Ancient Greek.* Culture Trip. https://theculturetrip.com/europe/greece/articles/how-to-eat-like-an-ancient-greek/

Dr. Mehmat. (n.d.). *What are the benefits of drinking Greek coffee? | Coffee & Health.* Sharecare. Retrieved December 22, 2021, from https://sharecare.com/health/coffee-drink-health/what-benefits-drinking-greek-coffee

Greek olive oil: the history and the future of a multifaceted product. (n.d.). Greeknewsagenda.gr. Retrieved December 17, 2021, from https://greeknewsagenda.gr/topics/business-r-d/7335-greek-olive-oil-the-history-and-the-future-of-a-%E2%80%9Cblessed%E2%80%9D-product

greekmedicine.net. (n.d.). *Greek Medicine: HERBAL MEDICINE.* Www.greekmedicine.net. http://www.greekmedicine.net/therapies/Herbal_Medicine.html

Kotsiris, K. (2014, October 31). *Eating Like an Ancient Greek.* The Spruce Eats; TheSpruceEats. https://

www.thespruceeats.com/eating-like-an-ancient-greek-1705715

Liagre, L. (2021, January 28). *Horta*. 196 Flavors. https://www.196flavors.com/horta/

Moore-Pastides, P. (2010). *Greek revival : cooking for life*. University Of South Carolina Press.

OliveTomato. (2012, September 28). *Food and Diet: Ancient Greece vs. Modern Greece*. Olive Tomato. https://www.olivetomato.com/food-and-eating-ancient-greece-vs-modern-greece/

Petrovska, B. B. (2012). Historical review of medicinal plants' usage. *Pharmacognosy Reviews*, *6*(11), 1. https://doi.org/10.4103/0973-7847.95849

Radinovsky, L. (n.d.). *The History of Olive Oil in Greece*. Greek Liquid Gold: Authentic Extra Virgin Olive Oil. https://www.greekliquidgold.com/index.php/en/olive-oil-info/the-history-of-olive-oil-in-greece

Rahal, A., Kumar, A., Singh, V., Yadav, B., Tiwari, R., Chakraborty, S., & Dhama, K. (2014, January 23). *Oxidative Stress, Prooxidants, and Antioxidants: The Interplay*. BioMed Research International. https://www.hindawi.com/journals/bmri/2014/761264/

Rosenthal, E. (2008, September 24). Flood of junk food puts Greeks at risk. *The New York Times*. https://www.nytimes.com/2008/09/24/world/europe/24iht-diet.1.16435791.html

Team, G. (2020). *Why a Greek diet is considered Best in the world*. Greek City Times. https://greekcitytimes.com/2018/05/03/why-a-greek-diet-is-considered-best-in-the-world/

The Science Behind Greek Food's Amazing Healthy Properties. (2021, July 4). GreekReporter.com. https://greekreporter.com/2021/07/04/science-greek-food-healthy/

Wikipedia Contributors. (2019, November 13). *Ancient Greek cuisine*. Wikipedia; Wikimedia Foundation. https://en.wikipedia.org/wiki/Ancient_Greek_cuisine

ABOUT THE AUTHOR

Yota Kouyas Gerrior R.H.N is an emerging author of Holisitc Health & Wellness Practices. For ten years, Yota has been researching and studying ways to improve her overall health and wellness. After studying at CSNN, The Canadian School of Natural Nutrition, she decided to start a series of books to share her findings with others; In hopes that she can help them find ways to improve their overall health and wellness. This is her second book. If you liked this book, she would be grateful for a review on Amazon. You might also be interested in learning more about Yota's Holistic health and wellness practices. Look for her first book on Amazon called "Holistic Health with Nutrition: A Simple 11 Step Approach to Holistic Health with Nutrition".

ALSO BY
YOTA KOUYAS GERRIOR R.H.N

Holistic Health & Nutrition

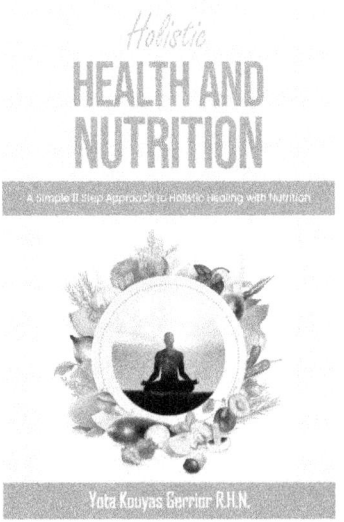

A Simple 11 Step Approach to Holistic Healing with Nutrition

www.ingramcontent.com/pod-product-compliance
Lightning Source LLC
Chambersburg PA
CBHW031153020426
42333CB00013B/651